Parenting Guide to Raising ADHD Boys

Contents

Chapter One

Introduction

Introduction

Hello and welcome to a journey that is as personal as it is universal – the journey of parenting boys with ADHD. My name is Patrick J Steadman, and I'm not just the book's author; I am a fellow traveler on this complex and often misunderstood path. I have raised seven children and one granddaughter raised as Our daughter, three of whom have ADHD, and have witnessed firsthand the profound impact this condition can have on their lives – from lost relationships and destructive behaviors to the daily struggles and intense confrontations that come with it. Please forgive me for the humor. Sometimes, if you don't laugh, you'll cry. Nobody has ever asked me to lighten up, so I hope you can enjoy reading.

This book is born out of my desire to share these life experiences – successes and challenges. It reflects my journey, from the moments of deep frustration to the times of incredible triumph. My motivation is rooted in showing you, the reader, the possibilities within the struggles and sharing the success stories that often go untold.

One of my sons, living with ADHD and dyslexia, often found himself lost in his world during class, gazing out the window while embarking on imaginative adventures in his mind. These experiences, while challenging, have also opened up a world of understanding and empathy.

Our approach in navigating these waters has been to seek answers from two realms – the spiritual wisdom found in Biblical teachings and the empirical evidence provided by scientific studies on ADHD. This dual approach has been our compass, guiding us through the complexities of ADHD parenting.

On these pages, you'll find a guide and a companion. This book combines personal anecdotes, biblical insights, and the latest scientific information on ADHD. It's designed to offer you a holistic understanding of your child, going beyond the conventional advice to explore deeper, more meaningful strategies for nurturing and guiding your ADHD boy.

This book is for you, whether at the beginning of this journey or well on your way. It's for every parent who has watched their child struggle and yearned to make a difference. Together, we will explore how to turn challenges into growth, strength, and success opportunities.

Join me in this journey, and let's discover the extraordinary potential that lies within our extraordinary boys.

Warm regards,

Patrick J Steadman

Chapter Two

Strengthening Parent-Child Bonds

Importance of Emotional Connection

As we begin on this journey, don't worry. I'm not a Bible thumper; certain bible verses sometimes really can speak to our issues, though. In the journey of parenting a child with ADHD, the cornerstone is undoubtedly the emotional connection between parent and child. This bond is the lifeline through which we can guide, understand, and support our children. It's essential to recognize that children with ADHD often experience a world that is overwhelming and confusing, which can lead to emotional outbursts and frustrations. Our role as parents is to provide a stable, understanding, and empathetic environment where they feel safe and loved.

The Mama Bear: Advocacy and Understanding in the School System

My wife has been a pillar of strength in our family's journey with ADHD. Affectionately known as the 'Mama Bear,' she has tirelessly fought for understanding and support within the school system. Her advocacy began in earnest when we first encountered challenges with our son's behavior at school. These were trying times, with our son experiencing aggressive outbursts and deep-seated frustrations symptomatic of his yet-to-be-diagnosed ADHD.

Diagnosis and Collaboration: A Turning Point

The turning point came with his diagnosis, made possible through the collaboration of his physician, teachers, other educational professionals, and, yes, Mama Bear. This diagnosis was not merely a label but a gateway to understanding. It opened doors to resources and strategies that were previously unavailable or unknown to us. It was a moment of validation and recognition of the struggles our son had been silently enduring.

Practical Strategies for Building Trust and Understanding

Once we understood the 'why' behind our son's behavior, we could implement practical strategies that made a real difference.

Creating Social Contracts:
We worked with our son to develop social contracts. These agreements, co-created with him, outlined acceptable behaviors and pro-

vided a clear structure for him to understand the consequences of his actions.

- Consistent Routines: Establishing predictable routines helped our son feel more secure and in control of his environment. Homework as soon as he got home from school; waiting for later means never. The funny thing is that our dog did eat his homework once. It took a little convincing, but we fully believed after we found our pups' deposits in the yard. ADHD kids suffer from such disorganized thoughts. You need a list for them to follow, preferably with checkboxes, as they complete the tasks, and if the parent has ADHD, you'll need one to make sure you look at the list.

- Open Communication: We encouraged open and honest communication in our household, ensuring our son knew he could express his feelings without fear of judgment. But with less cursing, the better for Papa Bear.

- Positive Reinforcement: We focused on his strengths, celebrating small victories and positive behaviors, which helped boost his self-esteem, such as not fighting with his siblings and or getting stabbed by anyone for a later chapter.

- Parental Patience and Empathy: Perhaps most importantly, we learned the value of patience and empathy. Understanding that our son's actions were not willful disobedience but rather manifestations of his ADHD changed our perspective entirely.

This chapter of our lives has been a journey of learning and adaptation. It has taught us the power of emotional connection and the importance of advocating for our children's needs. Through patience, understanding, and perseverance, we have strengthened our bonds and laid a strong foundation for our son to grow and thrive. I didn't simply want this to be a book of facts, but it to be a book of our travels and some of the things we found, even the difficult things. But our society in the past and sometimes, even today, look at parents with ADHD children as having done something wrong with the way they raised them; this isn't true. I know that our lives, flawed as they may be, are not any worse than anyone else's. That's my opinion anyway. As I look back, it's not simply with an understanding of the data, the findings, and the science but of our love for one another and how our many struggles have given us a strength that no amount of knowledge could ever do. So, let's move on before I cry.

As our understanding deepened, so did our approach to parenting. We realized that the emotional connection with our child is about responding to behaviors and proactively building a relationship based on trust, understanding, and mutual respect. Here are some additional strategies that we found exceptionally compelling:

Fostering Emotional Intelligence

We encouraged our son to recognize and express his feelings. This self-awareness is crucial for children with ADHD, as it helps them understand their emotional triggers and learn how to manage them. We always heard something like they made me mad. That's why I screamed at them. Or if "they didn't act that way, I wouldn't act this way." It was a clever mantra, but it did not affect us. How to address disobedience will be addressed later in this book.

As parents, we aimed to model calm and composed behavior, especially in challenging situations. So, this was not always the case.

Sometimes, you ran around in a circle like your hair was on fire. But when we acted calmly, we got much better responses. It isn't easy to be as perfect as we are (I'm kidding!). This helped our son learn, by example, how to regulate his emotions. This was not always successful, and sometimes, I wanted to pull my hair out, so my wife came over to help me. Pull my hair out, I mean. And I helped her by holding both hands over my ears until the fussing was over. Somehow, we didn't think that was the best technique, so I tried to pay attention as much as possible. I told her I had an attention deficit, too, but she didn't believe me.

Learning to Listen

We practiced active listening, which involves fully concentrating, understanding, responding, and remembering what is being said. My problem was remembering. I knew she said something, but I wasn't sure what it was the next day, and she filed all my forgettance away, for our later arguments, it's a talent; I couldn't contend with her. Practicing active listening helped our son feel heard and allowed us to understand his perspective better. We made it a point to validate his feelings, regardless of how trivial they might seem. This validation helped him feel respected and valued. Sometimes, his feelings may have been a little quirky. But I validated him as (the family's great father and Papa Bear). My mother was a child of German immigrants of a family of 12, not including Grandpa and Grandma. Germans in the 1980s were somewhat stoic and not so affectionate, so for me, this was a big learning curve. My sons would hug their friends and have their arms on each other's shoulders when they walked. I didn't have a problem with it, But as an adult male, I felt a little uncomfortable hugging other adult males. When I became more enlightened, I now hug all my children. But not My friends. Let's move on.

Collaborative Problem-Solving

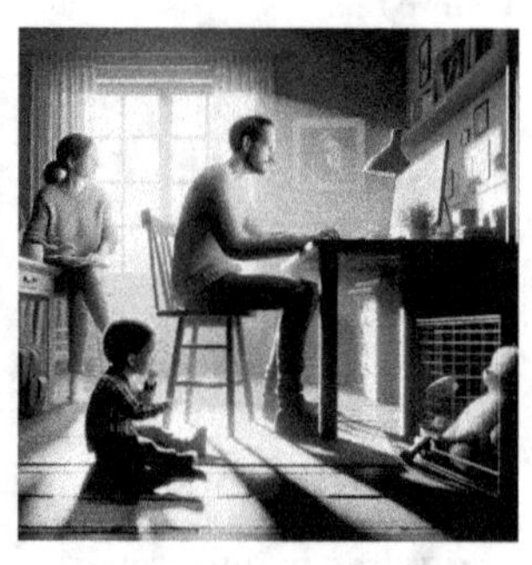

We involved our son in decisions that affected him, especially his ADHD. This inclusion gave him a sense of control and responsibility. When is-sues arose, we sat down as a family to brainstorm solutions. This collaborative approach fostered a sense of teamwork and made our son feel like an active participant in managing his ADHD.

Celebrating Uniqueness

We embraced our son's unique perspective and talents, celebrating the positives of ADHD, such as his creativity and out-of-the-box think-ing. We educated ourselves extensively about ADHD and also took the time to educate family members, friends, and educators about it. This created a more supportive and understanding environment for our son.

The Role of Faith and Science

A blend of faith and scientific understanding guided our journey. The biblical principles provided us with patience, hope, and the strength to face challenges, while scientific studies on ADHD offered practical insights and strategies to implement. This holistic approach was instrumental in not just managing the symptoms of ADHD but in nurturing a well-rounded individual.

Navigating the Highs and Lows

Parenting a child with ADHD is akin to navigating a ship in ever-changing seas. There are calm, serene days filled with profound joy and pride. And then, there are stormy days marked by frustration and misunderstandings. Through it all, we've learned the importance of remaining steady and resilient, using each experience as a learning opportunity. Rigidity often backfires with children who have ADHD. We learned to be flexible, adapting our approaches as needed. This flexibility allowed us to respond more effectively to our son's changing needs. We surround ourselves with people who understand and support our family's journey. This network included other parents of children with ADHD, healthcare professionals, and empathetic friends and family. We didn't always concern ourselves about everybody knowing everything about ADHD; it just seems a little Karen-ish.

Building a Toolbox of Strategies

Just as no two children with ADHD are the same, no single strategy works for all. We built a toolbox of diverse approaches, picking and choosing what worked best for our son in different situations. From reward systems, i.e., charts with stickers to time-outs, we experimented with various behavioral techniques, always focusing on positive reinforcement and clear, consistent communication. My favorite is that once your child is a teen, give them a phone you control, such as when and how they use it. I used to cut their phones off all the time when they were acting incorrectly. This created some crazy situations in our home, but it was worth it overall. We are watching a teen meltdown. I think you know what I mean. We worked closely with our son's school to ensure he had the accommodations to succeed academically, such as extra time on tests or a quiet place to study. Health and Wellness: We paid close attention to diet, exercise, and sleep – all of which significantly impact ADHD symptoms. Ensuring a healthy lifestyle was a crucial part of our strategy.

The Journey Continues

As our son grows and evolves, so do our strategies and understanding. What remains constant is our unconditional love and commitment to his well-being. Our journey is ongoing, and each day brings new challenges and triumphs.

Chapter Three

Understanding ADHD and Its Impact on Boys

No victory is too small to celebrate. Whether it's a successful day at school or managing to control an emotional outburst, we celebrate these moments, reinforcing positive behaviors and achievements. Our journey with ADHD is as much a learning experience for us as it is for our sons. We continue to educate ourselves and stay abreast of the latest research in ADHD and child development.

ADHD Symptoms Specific to Boys

In our journey to understand ADHD, it's crucial to recognize how it uniquely affects boys. Boys are often diagnosed with ADHD more frequently than girls, and

the symptoms can manifest differently, influencing their behavior, learning, and social interactions.

Hyperactivity in Boys

Hyperactivity in boys with ADHD often presents as a nearly constant state of motion. They might fidget, tap, or find it hard to sit still. This restlessness is often most noticeable in structured environments like the classroom, where their need for movement can be misinterpreted as disruptive behavior. Ephesians 6:4 cautions us as parents to be mindful in our approach, especially when dealing with a child's hyperactivity, which can often be frustrating. We must remain patient and avoid projecting our frustrations onto the child, ensuring we support them with understanding and compassion. I'm sure the Torah and the Quran have similar messages.

Impulsivity and Risk-Taking

Impulsivity in boys with **ADHD** can lead to actions without considering the consequences. This trait often manifests in risk-taking behaviors and challenges with self-control, which can be particularly stressful in social and school settings.

Inattention in boys with **ADHD** might look like daydreaming, difficulty following instructions, or seeming not to listen when spoken to directly. This can significantly impact their academic performance, as they might struggle to focus on tasks or organize their work. Early in my 20s, after I was discharged out of the army, where I was a medic. I opened a construction business, and my son occasionally worked with me when he was not 8 or 9, helping pick up scrap. I showed him how to pick up the scrap pieces off the floor, put them in the wheelbarrow, and bring them to the window. He was shown where to throw them out into a dumpster. Whenever I returned to the room, he would be on the floor making pyramids with the pieces of drywall or hammering nails with his shoe. Then I realized I would have to find something else for him to do. At that time, I didn't need a small pyramid builder.

The intersection of ADHD and Dyslexia

My son's story isn't just about ADHD; it's also about navigating the complexities of dyslexia, a learning disorder characterized by difficulties in reading. The co-occurrence of ADHD and dyslexia is not uncommon, yet it presents a unique set of challenges. Studies have shown that children with both ADHD and dyslexia may have more severe difficulties in academic achievement and self-esteem. The struggle to focus and the challenge of decoding words can make learning an exhausting task for these children. They didn't study my boy with ADHD and dyslexia. He had great self-esteem, in fact, almost too much.

Real-Life Impact: A Personal Story

A poignant example of how ADHD symptoms can escalate occurred during a basketball game involving my son. His inability to control his impulses led to an aggressive outburst on the basketball court, suspending him. This incident was a stark reminder of how ADHD can impact not just academic but also social and extracurricular activities. After he was pulled from that game, getting along with the other boys on the team became very difficult, leading him to no longer want to play. It was unfortunate for him and all of us. He was really good. I felt he could have played college ball. This broke my heart for him. I wish I could have forced him to return to the team, but it was impossible after speaking to his coach, who said he couldn't manage his behavior. ADHD in the 1980s was not well understood, but at first, I felt I wanted to punch his coach. But that would set us a bad example, and he would have beaten me up. He was a huge guy. "Just being honest". Inattention in boys with ADHD might look like daydreaming, difficulty following instructions, or seeming not to listen when spoken to directly. This can significantly impact their academic performance, as they might struggle to focus on tasks or organize their work.

In academics, boys with ADHD often struggle with maintaining focus during lessons and organizing tasks. Behavioral challenges frequently arise from difficulty managing emotions and adhering to expected social norms. Like laughing at someone when they trip and fall, even if it was his father. Meanie. Inattention in boys with ADHD might look like daydreaming, difficulty following instructions, or seeming not to listen when spoken to directly. And trust me, louder doesn't work. This can significantly impact their academic performance, as they might struggle to focus on tasks or organize their work.

"Children are great imitators. So give them something great to imitate, but don't be surprised when
they repeat everything you shouldn't have said in
the first place. "

Chapter Four

The impact of ADHD on boys extends beyond the individual symptoms;

Learning, Behavior, and Socialization in Boys with ADHD in the next chapter

Case Study: Classroom Incident

A notable incident that further illustrates these challenges happened in my son's classroom. He was passing a note, a common enough activity in schools, but when the teacher intercepted it, his reaction was swift and physical – he grabbed her arm. Who knew this was a crime? After the incident, she said she felt intimidated, so I understood this was wrong behavior, and we went to court.   At first, this was not a very good disciplinary action for me, but after the judge read him the riot act, this allowed me to get him to do chores for at least a week. This impulsive reaction, a direct result of his ADHD, led to a suspension and highlighted the need for constant vigilance and understanding from educators and parents alike.

Behavioral Dynamics in Family and School

In families, the behavioral dynamics can shift dramatically with an ADHD diagnosis. Parents often have to adopt new roles, sometimes acting as advocates, teachers, or counselors. The need for consistent discipline paired with understanding and support becomes paramount.

In school, these boys may often feel misunderstood. Traditional educational environments aren't always equipped to handle the unique needs of children with ADHD. Their behaviors, frequently misinterpreted as defiance or lack of interest, can lead to punitive measures, such as in the case of my son's suspension, rather than supportive interventions.

Social Challenges and Misunderstandings

Socially, boys with ADHD can face significant challenges. They might struggle with making and keeping friends, often due to misunderstandings of their behavior. Their impulsivity can be off-putting to peers, and their hyper-activity can be overwhelming in social settings.

ADHD, Dyslexia, and the Learning Curve

The combination of **ADHD** and dyslexia presents a complex learning curve. My son's mind was always on the go, filled with creative thoughts and ideas. Yet, the structure of traditional learning environments and the challenge of dyslexia made academic achievement particularly difficult. Understanding and navigating this intersection became a key focus for us as parents.

Emotional Toll and Building Resilience

The emotional toll on boys with **ADHD** can be significant. Feelings of frustration, low self-esteem, and anxiety are common. For my son, his outbursts were physical reactions and emotional expressions of his inner turmoil. Building emotional resilience became a crucial aspect of our parenting approach.

Strategies for Emotional Regulation

- **Encouraging Expressive Activities:** Art, music, or sports can provide a constructive outlet for emotions and energy.

- **Creating Safe Spaces for Conversation:** Establishing a judgment-free zone at home where feelings can be expressed and discussed openly.

- **Teaching Relaxation Techniques:** Deep breathing or

mindfulness can help manage emotional responses.

Advocacy and Empathy: Keys to Success

Through our experiences, we learned that advocacy and empathy are indispensable tools in the journey of parenting a boy with ADHD. Advocacy involves fighting for your child's rights and educating those around him – teachers, relatives, and peers – about the nuances of ADHD.

Ephesians 6:4 advises that our role as parents is not to exacerbate our children's challenges but to nurture them with kindness. This approach not only sets a positive example but also demonstrates the behaviors and values expected of them.

Empathy is about truly understanding the world from your child's perspective. It's about acknowledging their struggles and celebrating their unique way of experiencing life.

Understanding the full spectrum of ADHD's impact is crucial for developing effective parenting strategies. It's not just about managing the symptoms; it's about nurturing a child who sees and interacts with the world differently.

Nurturing Independence and Confidence

A key aspect of parenting boys with ADHD is fostering a sense of independence and confidence. Due to their unique challenges, these children often face more criticism and negative feedback, which can erode their self-esteem. Focus on identifying and nurturing their strengths and interests. This can be a powerful way to boost their confidence and self-esteem. Offering tasks and activities that are challenging yet achievable can help them develop a sense of accomplishment. We suffered the boomerang effect for the longest time of our kids when they left home and came back until We purchased a smaller house, not really.

The next chapter is even more exciting than this chapter, so curl up in a good chair, and let's read on.

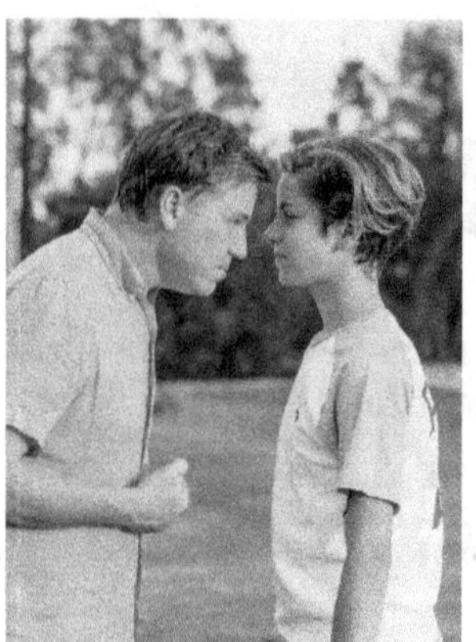

Anger control, careful to
manage ours and theirs

Individualized Learning Plans, Diet and Dealing with Specific behavior issues (Triggers)

Academic Adjustments and Support:

For children with ADHD and dyslexia, traditional academic methods often fall short. It becomes essential to tailor the learning experience to their specific need. They are working with educators to develop an Individualized Education Plan (IEP) that caters to their unique learning styles. The IEP makes a difference with ADHD kids and many kids in general who need a little more time to focus on the material and test-taking, etc. This is a great tool. They use technology and tools to aid learning in children with ADHD and dyslexia. For example, audiobooks can be an excellent resource for children who struggle with reading. My son and I often share audiobook recommendations; now that he's older, I enjoy it with him.

The Role of Physical Activity

Physical activity can play a significant role in managing ADHD symptoms. For my son, participating in sports was a double-edged sword d. While it provided an outlet for his energy, the structured environment of team sports sometimes clashed with his ADHD traits. Finding the right balance and the correct type of physical activity is complex. Individual or less structured team sports can sometimes be more suitable for children with ADHD. Regular physical activity can help manage energy levels and improve concentration. One of the things I did when they were little was have running competitions where usually the oldest would win, but since I could outrun them all, I got involved, and victory was mine. I told him, "You can't all win". I'm kidding, kind of.

Dealing with Behavioral Episodes

Behavioral episodes, such as the incidents on the basketball court and in the classroom, require a nuanced approach. Punitive measures alone are often ineffective and can exacerbate frustration and isolation. When my son was a baby, he repeatedly touched things he wasn't supposed to, like his sister. He couldn't help himself no matter what we did or how much we disciplined him; he would never give up the stereo, so finally, I had to put it up higher to keep him from touching it, and he tried to climb and get it. You got to give it to him. That's perseverance, anyway. Identifying what triggers these episodes, like cussing on the court, can be crucial in preventing them and working with the child to understand the consequences of their actions and to develop alternative responses.

Building a Supportive Community

Parenting a child with ADHD isn't a journey to be undertaken alone. Building a community of support is essential. This community can include family members, teachers, healthcare professionals, and parents of other children with ADHD. I also found encouraging responsible young people to hang out with my son; I made it known if he had a friend, a kid I didn't like, or felt he was trouble. As the Bible says, good company makes good morals. Sharing experiences and strategies with other parents can provide valuable insights and support. Regular consultations with professionals specializing in ADHD can give guidance and reassurance.

> Continuing with the theme of holistic approaches to managing ADHD, an important aspect to consider is the role of physical activity and exercise in mitigating ADHD symptoms.

The Power of Exercise in ADHD Management

The connection between physical activity and improved cognitive function in children with ADHD is increasingly supported by research. A study published in the *Journal of Abnormal Child Psychology* found that regular physical activity significantly improved attention and reduced impulsivity in children with ADHD. This aligns with our experiences where structured physical activities have offered a productive outlet for excess energy and helped improve focus and behavior.

- Structured Physical Activities: Activities like martial arts, swimming, or yoga, which require focus and discipline, can be particularly beneficial for children with ADHD.

- **<u>Consistency is Key:</u>** Regular engagement in physical activities is more effective than sporadic participation.

Behavioral Episodes and Physical Activity

Reflecting on the behavioral episodes, such as the basketball court incident, I recognize the importance of finding a suitable physical activity that aligns with a child's interests and ADHD symptoms. For some children with ADHD, competitive team sports might trigger anxiety or impulsive reactions. In contrast, individual sports or activities that emphasize personal growth and self-discipline might be more beneficial. Experimenting with different activities is important to find what best suits your child's temperament and interests. Engaging with empathetic and knowledgeable coaches who understand the unique needs of children with ADHD can make a significant difference.

Building Life Skills Through Exercise

The benefits of exercise extend beyond just physical health. They can play a crucial role in developing life skills such as teamwork, perseverance, and goal-setting. These skills are precious for children with ADHD, who often face challenges in these areas. Participating in team sports or group activities can help develop social skills and learn teamwork symptoms dynamics. Setting and achieving physical goals can boost self-esteem and a sense of accomplishment.

Beyond Physical Activity: Holistic Well-being

While physical activity is a crucial component, it's part of a larger picture of holistic well-being. My son suffered from insomnia from a young age, as did my stepson. We tried melatonin, but it had a lingering effect. Finding out what works for your child is sometimes as simple as a glass of warm milk. Nutrition, sleep, and mental health are equally important in managing ADHD. A balanced diet, adequate sleep, and mindfulness practices like meditation can complement physical activity to provide comprehensive support for children with ADHD.

As we navigate the complex world of ADHD, it becomes clear that there is **no one-size-fits-all** solution. Each child is unique, and our approaches must be tailored to their need. We can guide our children toward success and well-being through empathy, understanding, and strategic interventions like exercise.

Continuing with the holistic approach, let's delve deeper into the role of diet in managing ADHD and explore how specific foods and eating habits can impact behavior and cognitive function. Research has increasingly highlighted the connection between nutrition and the management of ADHD symptoms.

The Research on Diet and ADHD

Numerous studies have pointed to the potential impact of diet on ADHD symptoms.

For instance, Reduced Symptoms of Inattention after (Dietary Omega-3 Fatty Acid Supplementation in Boys with ADHD). Dienke J Bos et al. Neuropsychopharmacolog . 2015 Sep.

Building a Brain-Healthy Diet

Creating a diet that supports brain health can be a crucial component in managing ADHD. This involves incorporating foods rich in essential nutrients and avoiding those that might exacerbate symptoms. Omega-3-rich foods like salmon, tuna, and flaxseeds, high in omega-3 fatty acids, can benefit brain health. Whole Grains: Incorporating whole grains can help maintain stable blood sugar levels, which can be necessary for managing mood and energy. Fruits and Vegetables: A diet high in fruits and vegetables ensures adequate intake of essential vitamins and minerals.

A Recipe for Success

To illustrate how diet can be integrated into everyday life, here's a simple, nutritious recipe that is both kid-friendly and rich in brain-healthy nutrients:

Omega-3 Rich Salmon Patties

Ingredients:

- 2 cans of wild-caught salmon (drained)

- 1 beaten egg

- 1/2 cup whole grain breadcrumbs

- Two tablespoons finely chopped onion

- One tablespoon chopped fresh dill

- Salt and pepper to taste

- Olive oil for cooking

Instructions:

- Mix the salmon, egg, breadcrumbs, onion, dill, salt, and pepper in a bowl.

- Form the mixture into small patties.

- Heat olive oil in a pan over medium heat.

- Cook the patties on each side for 4-5 minutes or until golden brown.

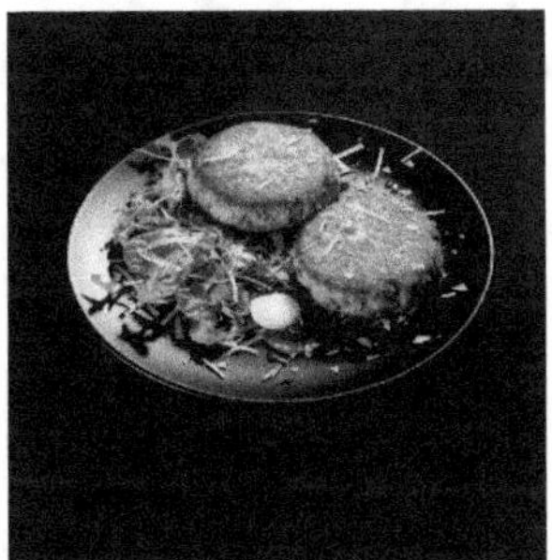

Serve these salmon patties with steamed vegetables or a fresh salad for a meal rich in beneficial nutrients for managing ADHD.

Avoiding Trigger Foods

While incorporating healthy foods, it's equally important to be aware of potential trigger foods. Some children with ADHD may be sensitive to certain food additives, sugars, and processed foods, which might exacerbate hyperactivity and attention issues. Our son found a sense of calm with stimulants, such as the caffeine in coffee. Interestingly, instead of increasing his hyperactivity, consuming a caffeinated beverage had the opposite effect, often leading him to become sleepy after periods of intense activity.

Continuing with the holistic management of ADHD, it's essential to understand that dietary adjustments are just one piece of a giant puzzle. Integrating these changes into a consistent lifestyle is critical to seeing meaningful improvements in ADHD symptoms.

Chapter Six

ADHD Medications, Self medicating and other Dietary things

S ome ADHD medications are stimulants, and caffeine, being a stimulant, can sometimes have similar effects. It may help improve concentration and focus for some individuals with ADHD. The effects of caffeine on ADHD symptoms can vary significantly from person to person. For some, it might improve focus and alertness, while for others, it could increase anxiety and exacerbate sleep issues. Caffeine would put one of our sons to sleep. Some individuals with ADHD use caffeine as a form of self-medication to help manage their symptoms. However, this should be approached cautiously, as caffeine can also have adverse side effects. Concerns About Overuse and Dependence: There's a risk of overuse or dependence on caffeine, mainly if it's being used regularly to manage ADHD symptoms. Excessive caffeine intake can lead to sleep disturbances, increased heart rate, and other health issues. Impact on Sleep: Individuals with ADHD often struggle with sleep, and caffeine can worsen these issues. It's essential to monitor caffeine intake and avoid it close to bedtime. Consultation with Healthcare Providers: Individuals with ADHD should consult with healthcare providers before using caffeine as a strategy to manage symptoms. A healthcare provider can offer guidance based on the individual's health history and specific symptoms. Research on the effects of caffeine on ADHD is ongoing, and there's still much to learn about how it affects different individuals.

Consistency and Routine in Diet

Consistency in dietary habits can be as important as the food choices themselves. Regular meal times and structured eating habits can provide the predictability and routine that children with ADHD often find reassuring. Structured Meal Times: Having fixed times for meals can help regulate the body's clock, which in turn can aid in managing ADHD symptoms. Healthy Snacking: Incorporating healthy snacks into the day can help maintain energy levels and stabilize mood, which is especially important for children with ADHD.

Involving Children in Meal Planning

Involving children with ADHD in meal planning and preparation can not only be a fun activity but also an educational one. It can teach them about nutrition, give them a sense of control, and encourage healthier eating habits. Use meal preparation as an opportunity to spend quality time together and educate about healthy food choices. Allowing children to make choices about their meals (within fit parameters) can empower them and make them more invested in their eating habits.

Monitoring and Adjusting

Just as every child with ADHD is unique, so is their response to different foods. It's essential to monitor how certain foods affect your child's behavior and adjust as needed.

- Food Journaling: Keeping a food diary can help identify correlations between diet and ADHD symptoms.

- Regular Reviews: Review and adjust the diet in consultation with healthcare professionals if necessary.

Beyond Diet: The Broader Lifestyle Approach

While diet is a critical component in managing ADHD, it's important to remember that it's most effective when combined with other lifestyle interventions. As discussed earlier, regular exercise is vital in managing ADHD symptoms.

- Sleep Hygiene: The importance of regular and sufficient sleep for children with ADHD is underscored by various scientific studies. Research has consistently shown that adequate sleep significantly influences behavior and attention spans in these children. Notably, studies link Obstructive Sleep Apnea (OSA) and children with (ADHD). These findings highlight the critical role of proper sleep hygiene in managing and potentially alleviating ADHD symptoms. Journal of Abnormal Child Psychology

- Mindfulness and Stress Reduction: Techniques for stress reduction and mindfulness can be particularly beneficial for emotional regulation and focus.

Drug use may simply be self-medicating or getting along with peers who are doing the same. I had one of my brothers, of which I had 4, and 4 sisters to match. "My parents like balance, I guess." He almost died from a drug overdose back in the '70s, being three years older than myself. He was able to instill fear early on in my life about drugs. This made me wonder what might happen if I touched non-prescribed medications so I could die. I seem to have taken it to heart because it came from him In a place of love.

Percentages of overdose deaths involving the most common opioids and stimulants alone or in combination[10] in 2022, *Overall (30 jurisdictions) CDC data 2022* SUDORS Dashboard: Fatal Overdose Data Final Data updated December 14, 2023; Preliminary Data updated December 14, 2023

Updated December 26, 2023

The five most frequently occurring opioids and stimulants, alone or in combination, accounted for **71.2% of overdose deaths**. The specific breakdown is represented below.

4.9% Cocaine with no other stimulants or opioids

6.2% Methamphetamine with no other stimulants or opioids

14.3% Illegally-made Fentanyl and Methamphetamine

17.5% Illegally-made Fentanyl and Cocaine

28.2% Illegally-made Fentanyls with no other opioids or stimulants

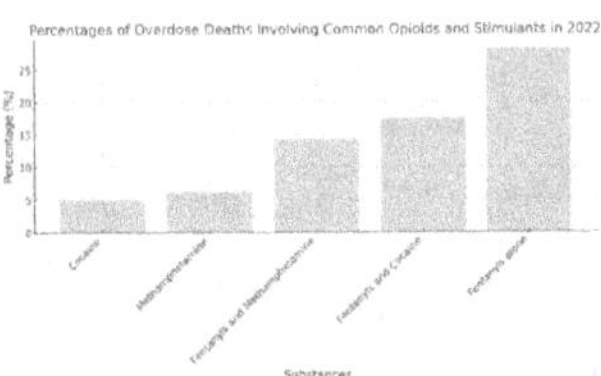

Okay, this may be boring to some, but I love data. I drooled over the CDC page. I'm a trained Six Sigma Black Belt. So I had to Kung Fu this unnecessary graph for you.

The dangers of overdose today for young people are higher than it's ever been, with the ease of access to opioids and stimulants attractive to ADHD kids and teens being epidemic. Today, parents need diligence in knowing who their children's friends are. Going through their backpacks, checking their computer and phone use, and looking for the signs of drug use are more important than ever before. In 2022, **per 100,000 people, 70 .5% who died of a drug overdose were male.**

Managing ADHD in children is a multifaceted challenge that requires a holistic approach. While diet plays a crucial role, it works best when integrated with a broader lifestyle strategy that includes physical activity, proper sleep, and emotional well-being. Through consistent, balanced, and mindful approaches, we can create an environment that supports the growth and development of children with ADHD, helping them academically and socially thrive.

As we move to the next part of this book, we'll explore specific behavioral management strategies and educational supports that can further aid in the journey of parenting a child with ADHD.

The journey of parenting a boy with ADHD is filled with challenges, but it is also a journey of immense growth and learning. It's about understanding and embracing how these children see the world. As we continue to explore this journey, remember that each step is a step toward building a resilient, confident, and happy child.

This chapter provides a glimpse into the multifaceted nature of ADHD in boys. The journey is not without its challenges, but with understanding, patience, and tailored strategies, these challenges can be transformed into opportunities for growth and development. As we progress in this book, we will explore specific strategies and approaches to help boys with ADHD thrive in all areas of their lives.

Chapter Seven

Creating a Supportive Home Environment

Creating a nurturing and structured environment at home is pivotal for children with ADHD. It's about building a space where they feel secure, supported, and capable of meeting their potential. This chapter focuses on structuring your home and establishing routines that can significantly aid in managing ADHD symptoms.

Structuring Your Home for Success

A well-structured home environment can provide the stability and predictability that children with ADHD need. This doesn't mean your home has to be a rigid, inflexible space, but rather an organized space that reduces distractions and encourages focus. If possible, create a specific area in the house for study and homework. This area should be free from distractions like TV and games. Keeping living spaces tidy and organized can help reduce the feeling of chaos, which can be overwhelming for children with ADHD. Tidiness comes with total family involvement. Make sure you have chore charts from an early age based on visual aids like calendars, color-coded systems, and labels that can help children understand and adhere to the organization of the home. Chores reflect a child's first responsibilities. We set our chart based on age and the standard expectations in the early years.

Establishing Routines and Expectations

Routines provide a sense of security and predictability for children with ADHD. They help set boundaries and expectations, which can be a comforting guide in their daily lives. Establish a daily routine that includes regular times for meals, homework, play, and bedtime. Clear Expectations: Communicate the expectations for behavior and daily tasks. Children with ADHD often benefit from knowing exactly what is expected of them. The Child Development Institute offers chare charts based on age available at https://childdevelopmentinfo.com/chores/the-ultimate-list-of-age-appropriate-chores/

**Example Schedule for a Young Boy with ADHD
Morning Routine**

- 7:00 AM: Wake up and morning hygiene

- 7:30 AM: Breakfast

- 8:00 AM: Prepare for school

- 8:30 AM: School or homeschooling activities

Afternoon Routine
- 3:00 PM: Snack and relaxation time

- 3:30 PM: Homework or educational activities

- 5:00 PM: Playtime or outdoor activities

Evening Routine
- 6:00 PM: Dinner

- 7:00 PM: Family time or quiet activities

- 8:00 PM: Bedtime routine starts

- 8:30 PM: Lights out

Example Schedule for a Teenager with ADHD

Morning Routine

- 6:30 AM: Wake up, shower, and personal hygiene

- 7:00 AM: Breakfast

- 7:30 AM: Prepare for school

- 8:00 AM: School or structured activities

Afternoon/Evening Routine

- 4:00 PM: Snack and downtime

- 4:30 PM: Homework or study time

- 6:00 PM: Extracurricular activities or exercise

- 7:30 PM: Dinner

- 8:30 PM: Free time or hobbies

Night Routine

- 9:30 PM: Start winding down, reduce screen time

- 10:00 PM: Bedtime routine

- 10:30 PM: Lights out

These are examples. Please adjust to your parenting practices. Of course, this is the perfect schedule, but you do you (kidding).

Building on the foundation of a structured and supportive home environment, we can delve deeper into the nuances of creating a space that not only supports the daily routines of children with ADHD but also fosters their emotional growth and learning.

Adapting the Home Environment for Different Needs

The needs of children with ADHD can vary significantly, and it's essential to tailor the home environment to meet these individual requirements. Quiet Zones vs. Active Areas: Some children may need a quiet, secluded space to retreat to when they feel overwhelmed, while others might benefit from areas where they can be active and expend energy. Sensory Considerations: For children sensitive to sensory inputs, having a space with minimized clutter, soft lighting, and calming colors can be beneficial. As I write this week, I have four grandkids and their mom living with us. My daughter asked last year if she could live with us until she gets on her feet. My attention deficit is leaving my head swimming at 63 years old.

How difficult could it have been for a child with ADHD? At one point, when all our seven children were home, two were under two years old, and the eldest was 18 years old. Could you imagine? While my wife and I were at work, the teenagers opened the second-story window and removed the screen. What then? Taking turns (at least they were taking turns) jumping out the window to land on the trampoline 20 ft below. Indeed, I would never have known about this if I hadn't just happened to come home while the perpetrators were in the action. Our eldest is up in her room on the phone. They didn't (I think) realize the additional height added thrust, sending them over the net or tangled.

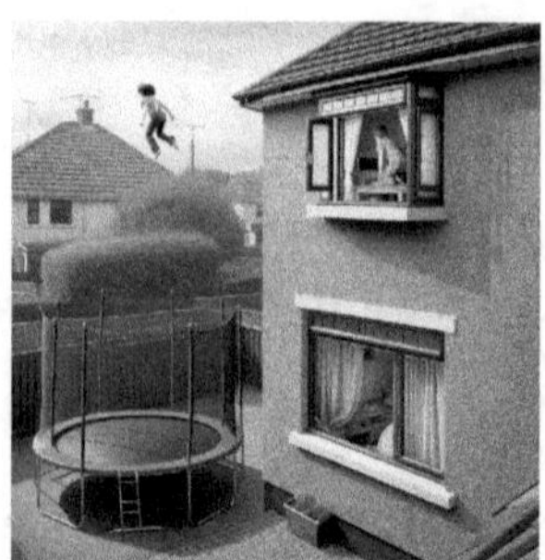

Bad choices

In it. When you have three children in the mix with ADHD, one was excused as she couldn't reach the window sill yet. I was amazed they didn't throw the baby out the window as She was standing s in line. Later that day, I drove screws into sills, not allowing them to open the window (a simple adaptation).

Involving Children in the Process

Involving children in organizing and structuring their space can empower them and give them a sense of ownership. This involvement can also provide valuable insight into what works best for them. Allow children to make decisions about organizing their space within reasonable limits. This can range from choosing the color scheme to deciding where to store their toys or books. Responsibility: Assign age-appropriate tasks and responsibilities related to maintaining their space. This teaches responsibility and helps them understand the importance of organization and routine.

Incorporating Flexibility

While structure is important, so is flexibility. Being too rigid can lead to frustration and resistance. Finding a balance provides structure and allows for changes and adjustments as needed.

- Flexible Routines: Have a basic routine but be open to

change based on the day's needs. For instance, if a child is having a tough day, it might be necessary to adjust the schedule to accommodate their state of mind.

- Choice within Structure: Provide options within the established routine. For example, offer a choice between two activities during their designated playtime.

Technology and ADHD

In today's digital age, managing technology is essential to creating a supportive home environment for children with ADHD. Balanced Screen Time: Set clear guidelines for screen time. While technology can be a valuable tool for learning and entertainment, balancing it with offline activities is crucial. Educational Tools: Utilize technology as an educational tool. Many apps and online resources are designed to aid learning and development in children with ADHD.

Cultivating a Home of Learning and Growth

The home environment should be a place of learning and growth, not just for academic skills but also for life skills. Life Skills Development: Incorporate activities that teach life skills, such as cooking, gardening, or basic home repairs. These can be tailored to suit the child's age and abilities. Encouraging Curiosity: Create an environment that promotes curiosity and learning. This could be through books, DIY projects, science kits, or art supplies. Creating a supportive home environment for a child with ADHD is a dynamic and ongoing process. It involves understanding your child's unique needs, providing structure and routines, and incorporating flexibility and choice. By doing so, we create a space that not only supports the daily challenges of ADHD but also fosters a sense of security, independence, and growth.

Creating a supportive home environment for children and teenagers with ADHD involves more than just physical space organization; it's about establishing routines, clear expectations, and a system that fosters independence and responsibility. By providing structure and predictability in their daily lives, we can help them navigate their world more easily and confidently.

Continuing with the theme of creating a supportive home environment, an essential aspect for children with ADHD is the educational setting. Homeschooling becomes a viable option for some families, offering a tailored educational approach that aligns with their child's unique needs and learning style.

Chapter Eight

Exploring the Homeschool Option

Homeschooling can provide a more personalized and flexible learning experience for children with ADHD. Parents can tailor the curriculum and teaching methods to their child's strengths and challenges.

- Customized Learning: Homeschooling enables you to customize the learning pace, style, and content. For children with ADHD, this might mean breaking lessons into smaller, more manageable segments or incorporating more hands-on learning experiences.

- Flexibility in Scheduling: Traditional school schedules can be challenging for some children with ADHD. Homeschooling allows for a more flexible schedule, accommodating when the child is most attentive and engaged.

Structuring a Homeschool Environment

Creating a structured yet flexible home school environment is critical. While it offers more freedom than traditional schooling, maintaining a certain level of structure is vital for children with ADHD.

Establish a specific area in the home for learning activities. This space should be free from distractions and conducive to concentration. Routine and Breaks: Establish a daily routine that includes regular breaks. Children with ADHD often benefit from shorter learning periods interspersed with physical activity or rest. Include activities that allow for movement and sensory exploration, which can be beneficial in maintaining focus and engagement.

Balancing Homeschooling with Socialization

One of the concerns about homeschooling is the potential lack of socialization opportunities. However, there are many ways to ensure homeschooled children receive ample social interaction.

- Extracurricular Activities: Enroll your child in extracurricular activities such as sports, arts, or clubs. This provides opportunities for socialization, physical activity, and exploration of interests.

- Homeschool Groups and Co-ops: Join local homeschool groups or co-ops. These can provide social interaction with peers and support and resources for parents.

- Almost 7% of Children in the United States are home-schooled and growing.

The Role of Parents and Caregivers in Homeschooling

Homeschooling a child with ADHD is a significant commitment and requires active involvement from parents or caregivers. Parental Involvement: As a homeschooling parent, you must be actively involved in planning, teaching, and monitoring your child's learning. Seeking services and Support: Take advantage of available resources, such as online homeschooling programs, educational materials, and support groups for guidance and assistance. Creating a supportive home environment extends into the realm of education. Homeschooling can be a beneficial option for some families with children who have ADHD, offering a personalized and adaptable educational experience. By carefully structuring the homeschool environment, providing opportunities for socialization, and committing to active involvement, parents can create a successful and fulfilling educational journey for their child. As we move forward, the following chapters will focus on specific strategies for behavioral management and academic support, building upon the stable foundation established at home.

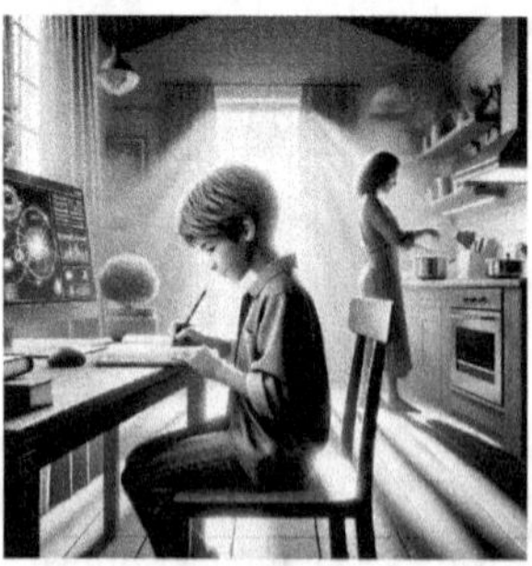

Chapter Nine

Behavior and Emotional Management

Effective Behavioral Management Techniques

In this chapter, we delve into the essential strategies for managing the behavior of children with ADHD. Effective behavioral management is not just about reducing unwanted behaviors; it's about nurturing positive habits, self-regulation, and emotional understanding. This chapter will explore techniques like positive reinforcement, discipline strategies, and methods to manage impulsivity and hyperactivity.

Positive Reinforcement and Discipline Strategies

Positive Reinforcement

The power of positive reinforcement in shaping a child's behavior cannot be overstated, especially for children with ADHD. It involves acknowledging and rewarding desired behaviors, which can encourage the child to repeat them. Immediate and Specific Praise: Offer praise immediately after the desired behavior occurs, and be specific about what you are praising. A reward system, such as a point or sticker chart, where accumulated points or stickers can be exchanged for a desired reward. Initially, we tried a system where they were allowed to cash in their stickers for money, but we soon found out that they didn't know the value of "coins"; we found quarters everywhere. It was an attempt to educate them about savings. This worked better when they were teenagers. Yet some teens don't know the value of money, and, unfortunately, adults even struggle with it. A better reward system is to have a present box and numbers on each item as to their value so they can buy them with their stickers. It worked well when we had young children. Maybe have teenagers earn games or phone time.

Discipline Strategies

Discipline for children with ADHD should be about teaching and guiding rather than merely pursuing it. The goal is to help them understand the consequences of their actions and learn to make better choices. Ensure that consequences for undesirable behavior are consistent and understood in advance by the child. **Time-Outs:** Use time-outs effectively, not as a punishment, but as an opportunity for the child to calm down and regain control. Engage in problem-solving with the child post-incident to discuss what happened and how to handle similar situations in the future.

Managing Impulsivity and Hyperactivity

Children with ADHD often struggle with impulsivity and hyperactivity, which can manifest in various ways, from interrupting conversations to acting without considering the consequences.

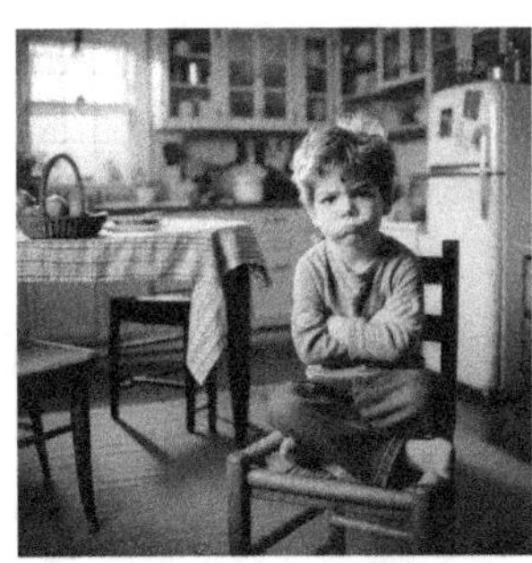

Every parent knows that face

Strategies for Impulsivity

Teach the child to take a moment to pause and think before acting. Role-playing different scenarios can be an effective way to practice this skill. Develop verbal cues or signals that you can use to remind the child to stop and think when you see them becoming impulsive.

Managing Hyperactivity

Provide regular opportunities for physical activity. Sports, dance, or even simple outdoor play can be effective ways for children to expend energy. During tasks that require focus, incorporate structured breaks where the child can get up, move around, and then return to the task. Continuing with the emphasis on behavioral and emotional management in children, let's further explore some advanced strategies and insights that can be particularly effective.

Advanced Strategies for Behavioral Management

In addition to the basic techniques, more nuanced strategies can be employed to manage and guide behavior in children with ADHD.

Setting Clear and Achievable Goals: Reduce significant goals into smaller, more manageable tasks. This can help the child feel a sense of achievement and progress. Use visual tools like charts or boards to track progress toward goals, which can motivate and reward the child. My granddaughter wanted a purple trash can (that's her favorite color) with a princess on it. My daughter told her that if she put money in her piggy, she'd eventually get enough to buy that trash can. It's so crucial that children see possibilities every time they go to the store's toy section. They should look at the toy they want and be told they can have it but must pay for it. "Stores don't give things away for free, little miss." One time, when we were still counting the months of our daughter's age, (I thought it would be better to use "1.534, 1.2565, months, etc." like a math problem). She grabbed the things she wanted when we weren't looking and threw them into her mother's basket. We took most of them out but unknowingly left one in the cart. This became a "huge crime" for our family. We used it as that annoying "teaching moment." She was escorted back to customer service to return her ill-gotten gains. She never did that again.

Cognitive Behavioral Techniques

Teach the child to use positive self-talk to combat negative thoughts and impulsive behavior. Develop their problem-solving skills through guidance. Activities and discussions help them think through the consequences of their actions.

Emotional Management and Regulation

Children with ADHD often experience intense emotions and may struggle with emotional regulation. Teaching them how to manage and express their feelings healthily is crucial.

Identifying and Expressing Emotions

Use games, charts, or storytelling to help the child identify and name different emotions. Encourage the child to express their feelings through words, art, or other creative outlets.

Relaxation and Calming Techniques

A child's simple breathing exercises can quickly and effectively calm down during moments of high emotion. Introduce mindfulness activities tailored to the child's age and interests, like guided meditations or yoga. Better still, teach them how to ride a bike.

Involving the Child in the Management Plan

Applying the child to help develop their behavior and emotional management plan can increase their engagement and commitment to the strategies. Please work with the child to create the behavioral plan, discussing what techniques they feel may work best for them. Discuss what's working and what isn't, and adjust the plan as needed.

Child 'As we continue to explore behavioral and emotional management, it's essential to consider the broader context of a child's life, including their educational environment and social interactions. These elements play a crucial role in the overall development and well-being of a child with ADHD.

Educational Support and ADHD

Navigating the educational system can be a challenge for children with ADHD. Tailored educational support is crucial in helping these children achieve their academic potential.

Collaboration with Educators

Open Communication: Establish open lines of communication with teachers and school staff to share insights about your child's needs and strategies that work well. IEP or 504 Plans: Work with the school to develop an Individualized Education Plan (IEP) or 504 Plan that outlines specific accommodations and support needed.

"We discovered that explaining to our children why they might need extra time can be helpful. Their unique minds process things differently, and understanding this can make things easier for them. While being pulled out of class might initially feel unsettling, the benefits far outweigh the initial discomfort."

At-Home Educational Strategies

Create a structured and distraction-free environment for homework and study. Educational Tools and Resources: Utilize tools and resources that cater to the child's learning style, such as interactive learning software or visual aids.

Social Interactions and ADHD

Social skills are often an area of difficulty for children with ADHD. Providing opportunities and support to help them develop these skills is essential to continue in the next chapter.

Chapter Ten

Life Skills, Faith and Emotional Intelligence

Social Skills Training

Use role-playing to practice social situations and responses, which can help the child feel more prepared for real-life interactions. Consider enrolling your child in social skills training groups where they can learn and practice skills in a structured environment. Choose extracurricular activities where your child can succeed and feel confident, which can foster positive peer interactions. Guide navigating social situations, including managing impulsivity and understanding social cues. As children with ADHD approach adolescence and adulthood, the focus of behavioral and emotional management shifts towards preparing them for the challenges of adult life.

Life Skills and Little Richey

Teach practical skills like budgeting, time management, and self-care, essential for independence. Plan for adulthood, including career planning and exploring post-secondary education options. Both of our sons, like many with ADHD, had disjointed plans as to what they wanted to do for a living. My wife's first husband was a plumber, and I feel that Richard was trying to have the relationship he always wanted with him, and that may have been why he became a plumber himself. My wife told me about how my stepson (I never use stepson; I use it here for identification purposes only. He is my son also). Like every young boy, Richard wanted a relationship with his father in early childhood and adulthood. They divorced when he was a child. When his father's visitation time would come up, he was supposed to pick him up at a scheduled time.

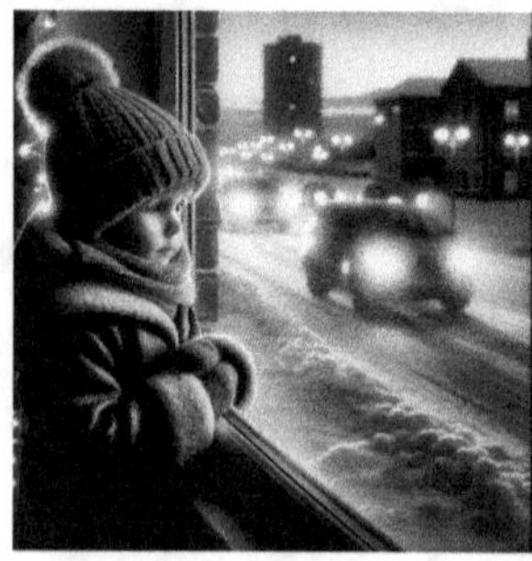

She told me he would stand at the window looking out into the street for 30 minutes," then an hour, then 2. With this coat, hat, and boots, waiting to leave. Excited to have this great day or the weekend with his father, after an hour or so, my wife would plead with him to remove his coat, sweat running down his cheeks mingled with tears. He would stand at the window indignant, jerking from her grasp, not wanting to miss any sign of the headlights approaching and after wife a couple of hours and watching neighbors' cars, waiting for his father to pull up. He curled up and cried himself to sleep, but before he did, "dosing off. He asked, "Wake me when he gets here". It's heartbreaking to think how tormented his young mind was; a boy who desires a relationship with a father who doesn't want one with him. It was all suited too not to lash out in front of him about his deadbeat father; okay, I said it. He didn't care if things were out of our control." Hi, honey, tostadas, you're the bestest wife ever." She came in while

I was dictating speech to text. Yes, I am that dorky, using baby talk with her. Again, don't tell anyone about this. I love my wife, and I love tostadas. Sue brought me the best tostadas I think I have ever eaten. Okay, now back to our journey

Mental Health and Well-being

Encourage open discussions about mental health and well-being, and seek professional help. Help the child build a network of friends, mentors, and professionals who can provide guidance and support. Too often, we overlook while helping our children to realize "that the apple didn't fall far from the tree." ADHD is our inheritance to our children. I'm sure you think that sounds crazy, but there are a lot of positive things about ADHD. It helps us succeed if we learn to channel it properly from childhood to adulthood. Like I said, my stepson, now a master plumber, makes a good living. But is still struggling with addiction. ADHD, in his case, can be such a massive burden, keeping him in that downward spiral yet helping him get his college degree. He feels he has to accomplish this independently, without help, like he did when he was young.   He has refused rehab or any other interventions. I came to this realization after years of battling and encouraging his financial and mental help. The little boy who stood at that window waiting for his father didn't see me when I arrived 23 years ago. He was fifteen years old when Sue and I married. I wish I had known him when he stood at that window; right, before we start crying, let's continue. We will ensure we have a sense of reality in this book. Not all children can escape bad choices made early in life. As we discussed earlier, addressing the fentanyl epidemic is essential.

Managing and supporting a child with ADHD is a multifaceted process that extends beyond the home into educational settings and social environments. By providing tailored academic support, fostering social skills, and preparing them for adulthood, parents can help their children with ADHD navigate these areas successfully. This holistic approach addresses immediate challenges and lays the foundation for a fulfilling and successful adult life.

"Effective behavioral and emotional management in children with ADHD is not a one-size-fits-all approach. It requires a combination of positive reinforcement, discipline strategies, emotional regulation techniques, and active involvement from the child. By employing a range of strategies and continuously adapting them to the child's evolving needs, parents can provide the support and guidance needed to help their child navigate The complexities of ADHD. This chapter focuses on the critical role of nurturing **emotional intelligence** in children with ADHD. Emotional intelligence is crucial to understanding, expressing, and regulating emotions effectively.

When I first heard the word emotional intelligence, I thought it was just more psychobabble that didn't mean anything. Many physicians and psychologists grasp the newest phrase or wordplay to define something. For boys with ADHD, who may face challenges with emotional regulation and sensitivity, I discovered these skills are even more crucial regardless of the words we use to define them. It's not just social interactions at play, but ADHD carries into every facet of their lives. Knowing your emotional state and how you express it to others with words or body language in a positive way can sometimes seem impossible. You're seated writing a book per se, and your beautiful grandchildren keep coming in to show you a picture, or so they've made. In my head, I want to snatch their face-off, but my reaction, controlled over years of vast experience, I stop for a minute and listen quietly, compliment them, and ask them not to come in so much, but I love seeing their work. I probably couldn't snatch their face off anyway. I'm not a chimpanzee. However, my wife might debate that somewhat.

Helping Your Son Understand and Express Emotions

Developing emotional intelligence, yes, there's that word again. It's growing on me. It begins with helping your son understand and healthily express his feelings. Use resources such as books, charts, and games to help your son learn about different emotions. (Or the thing about face snatching). Regularly discuss emotions and encourage your son to describe his feelings using specific terms.

Expressing Emotions Safely

Encourage activities like drawing, writing, or music to provide a safe and creative way for your son to express his motions. Demonstrate healthy ways of expressing emotions ourselves. Children often learn by observing their parents.

Techniques for Developing Resilience and Coping Skills

Resilience and coping skills are essential for children with ADHD to help them navigate life's challenges. Building resilience and working through problems together show that challenges can be overcome. This builds resilience. Praise efforts and resilience in the face of challenges, not just successes.

Developing Coping Strategies, Encouraging Self-Awareness and Empathy

Teach techniques such as deep breathing or mindfulness meditation to help manage stress and emotions. Use role-playing to practice coping strategies in different situations. We use the five-second rule or 10, having them count and take deep breaths before they answer or tell you what's happening. Occasionally, during the counting, they forgot what they were angry about and just stared out the window, waiting for a squirrel to pass by. A key aspect of emotional intelligence is understanding oneself and others.

Fostering Self-Awareness

Encourage regular times for reflection, helping your son to think about his actions and feelings. Writing about daily experiences and feelings can help increase self-awareness. Teaching Empathy talks about how others might feel in various situations and why. Engaging in community service or group activities can help your son understand and connect with the feelings of others. Volunteering somewhere that allows them to learn empathy as they serve others can build friendships.

Integrating a Faith Perspective in Emotional Development

Teaching Through Scripture

The Bible was the most excellent book ever written and sold more copies than any other book. Even if you're not a person of Faith, you can understand the value of the Bible's teachings. Other writings also have value from early authors, like the Torah and the Quran. Use stories and teachings from the early writings to illustrate healthy emotional expression and understanding. For example, the story of David can teach about managing fear and sadness. Encourage memorization of scriptures focusing on dynamic strength, empathy, and experience, like Philippians 4:13 or Colossians 3:12. Teach empathy and compassion through Jesus' example. Discuss how Jesus understood and cared for the emotions of others. Use biblical teachings to instill a sense of forgiveness and understanding, explaining that everyone makes mistakes and deserves compassion.

Applying Spiritual Teachings in Developing Resilience

Faith in Overcoming Challenges

Encourage prayer and reflection during difficult times, helping your son to turn to faith when facing emotional challenges. Share stories that demonstrate resilience, such as the story of Job or Paul, to inspire and teach perseverance. Engage with your worship community for support and guidance. Youth groups and places of worship activities can provide a sense of belonging and an environment to practice emotional intelligence skills. Involve your son in service and outreach opportunities through the place of worship, which can foster empathy and a sense of purpose.

Nurturing Emotional Intelligence: A Holistic Faith Approach

Whole-Person Development Emphasize the importance of spiritual, emotional, and mental development as they are interconnected in Faith teachings. Consider Faith counseling if additional support is needed, ensuring that emotional development aligns with your faith values. Incorporating a spiritual perspective into nurturing emotional intelligence adds spiritual depth and moral guidance. By integrating biblical teachings and faith values, we can provide our children a robust framework for understanding and managing their emotions. This approach not only addresses their needs as individuals with ADHD but also aligns with the spiritual and moral growth encouraged in Deuteronomy 6:7.

In the upcoming chapters, we will explore how these emotional and spiritual teachings can be integrated into broader life aspects, including education, social interactions, and family life.

Chapter Eleven

Educational Success and Social Skills

This chapter focuses on navigating the educational system for children with ADHD. This involves understanding how to effectively advocate for your child's needs in school and working collaboratively with teachers and educational professionals to ensure that your child receives the support and accommodations necessary for their success.

Advocating for Your Child in School

Understanding Your Child's Rights

- **Educate Yourself on Educational Laws:** Familiarize yourself with laws and policies such as the Individuals with Disabilities Education Act (IDEA) and Section 504 of the Rehabilitation Act. These laws provide for accommodations in the educational setting.

- **IEP and 504 Plans:** Learn about Individualized Education Programs (IEP) and 504 Plans, which are designed to provide support and accommodations for students with disabilities, including ADHD.

Effective Communication and Collaboration

Establish a positive and collaborative relationship with your child's teachers and administrators. Clear, open communication is critical. Schedule regular meetings with teachers to discuss your child's progress and any necessary adjustments to their educational plan.

Working with Teachers and Educational Professionals

Sharing Information and Insights

Share insights about how ADHD affects your child, including their strengths, challenges, and practical strategies that work at home. Engage in collaborative problem-solving with teachers to address academic or behavioral issues. Offer resources or suggest training opportunities for teachers on ADHD if needed. This can help them better understand and support your child. Recognize and appreciate the efforts of teachers and staff. Positive reinforcement can strengthen the collaborative relationship. Be your child's Mama or Papa Bear.

Building an Individualized Learning Plan

Tailoring Education to Your Child's Needs

Work with educational professionals to develop an individualized approach to your child's education, considering their unique needs and learning styles. Discuss specific accommodations that can support your child's learning, such as extended time on tests, reduced homework load, or the ability to take breaks when needed.

Authors Note

Navigating the educational system for a child with ADHD requires active involvement, advocacy, and collaboration. By understanding your child's rights, building strong relationships with school staff, and working to tailor your child's educational experience, you can help create an environment in which your child can thrive. Remember, you are your child's best advocate, and your involvement can significantly impact their educational journey.

Continuing with our exploration of navigating the educational system for children with ADHD, let's integrate a faith perspective, drawing inspiration from Deuteronomy 11:19 (KJV). This scripture emphasizes the importance of constant teaching and guidance, a principle that can be seamlessly applied to advocating for and supporting your child in their educational journey.

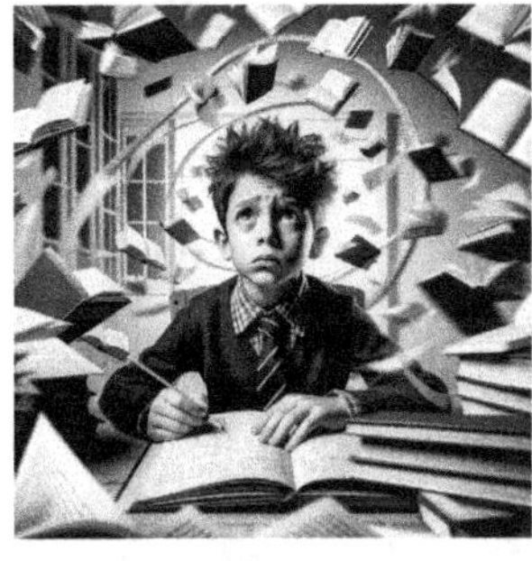

Integrating Faith Principles in Education

Teaching as a Continuous Process

Embrace the concept of teaching as an ongoing process. This can involve discussing educational topics and your child's school experiences in everyday situations, reinforcing the idea that learning isn't confined to the classroom. Incorporating Faith in Learning: Use opportunities to integrate faith and biblical teachings with academic learning, showing your child how their faith can guide and support them in their educational pursuits.

Moral Support and Guidance

Offer encouragement through scriptures, using them to motivate and comfort your child, especially when facing academic challenges. Demonstrate moral values such as patience, kindness, and perseverance in your interactions with educators and your approach to your child's education. Approach advocacy efforts with a Christ-like attitude, emphasizing love, respect, and understanding in your dealings with teachers and school administrators. Before meetings or discussions with school staff, seek guidance and wisdom to represent and support your child best.

Collaborating with Educators from a Faith Perspective

Building Relationships with Grace

Build relationships with your child's educators grounded in faith, practice, grace, and understanding to create a supportive and collaborative educational environment. Open Communication: Keep lines of communication open with teachers, sharing your child's progress and academic and spiritual challenges.

Integrating a Faith perspective into navigating the educational system involves more than just advocating for academic needs; it's about embedding biblical principles in every aspect of your child's education. By applying the teachings of Deuteronomy 11:19, you can create a holistic educational experience for your child that encompasses both academic knowledge and spiritual growth. This approach ensures that your child is supported intellectually and in their moral and spiritual development.

Continuing our exploration of navigating the educational system for children with ADHD from a Faith perspective, let's incorporate relevant statistics to provide a broader context and deepen our understanding of the challenges and opportunities in this area.

Understanding Through Statistics

Prevalence and Impact

Statistical Overview: According to the Centers for Disease Control and Prevention (CDC), approximately 9.4% of children in the United States between the ages of 2 and 17 have been diagnosed with ADHD, which translates to about 6.1 million children. This high prevalence underscores the importance of effective educational strategies. Academic Performance: Research indicates that children with ADHD are more likely to experience academic challenges. The National Center for Learning Disabilities reports that students with ADHD are three times more likely to drop out of school compared to their peers without ADHD.

Advocacy and Support: A Statistical Rationale

Importance of Advocacy

Access to Services: Studies show that early and consistent advocacy for children with ADHD leads to better access to educational services and accommodations. My stepson received an early diagnosis, and when we married in 2020, I realized that my 15-year-old son showed the same issues as his new brother. They came together as brothers. It was amazing. A report by the Child Mind Institute highlights that children who receive appropriate interventions are more likely to succeed academically and socially. Data suggests that parental involvement in education is a critical factor in the success of students with ADHD. A study published in the *Journal of Attention Disorders* found that students with ADHD whose parents were actively involved in their education had better outcomes in terms of grades and behavior. My wife was proactive in setting up meetings with teachers, always prepared to advocate firmly for our son's needs. The teachers knew we would promptly respond if they sent a note about his behavior. I often balanced the dynamic in these situations by adopting a more conciliatory approach, complementing my wife's assertiveness. This strategy enabled us to effectively address our child's needs, ensuring he received the support and guidance necessary for his development.

Integrating Faith Values: A Statistical Perspective

Faith and Academic Success

Impact of Faith on Education: While specific statistics on the intersection of faith and ADHD are limited, broader educational research suggests that a supportive environment, including spiritual support, positively influences academic achievement. For example, a study from Harvard University found that spiritual practices are associated with better mental and emotional well-being, which can contribute to academic success. Community Support: According to the Barna Group, children and teenagers who are part of a faith community tend to exhibit more vital social skills and higher engagement in school, indicating the potential positive impact of integrating Faith values in education for children with ADHD.

Homeschooling: Tailoring Education to Individual Needs
Personalized Learning Environment

Homeschooling allows parents to tailor the curriculum to fit their child's unique learning style, strengths, and challenges. Unlike traditional schools, homeschooling offers the flexibility to structure the day according to the child's most productive times.

Homeschooling allows parents to tailor the curriculum to fit their child's unique learning style, strengths, and challenges. Unlike traditional schools, homeschooling offers the flexibility to structure the day according to the child's most productive times.

•

Chapter Twelve

School Choice and Vouchers: Expanding Educational Opportunities

Homeschooling requires a significant time commitment from parents and a need for educational resources and planning. Parents must seek alternative ways to ensure their child receives adequate social interaction, such as through sports teams, clubs, or homeschooling. I was in my 20s with my former wife, and we had three children. This is not a religious book, But faith should not be ignored in our journey. If organized religion is not you, you may consider something as simple as meditation with you and your child, teaching them to tap into something more significant than the child.

Prayer for me has been a source of meditation, taking time to look outside myself and focus on how I might help others, Interceding to a higher power for my children's children. I also had a lot of help from our place of worship. After moving out of the area, the children were homeschooled using packets I purchased from a commercial home-teaching organization, which put them far ahead of the other children when I sent them to public school. The environment made a significant difference in their early lives and how they saw the world, and through my sons' ADHD, crazy bad ADHD, mind you. He was a massive challenge for my new wife, "New wife, that sounds kind of rude; she better not read this," she brought her son to the marriage, who had ADHD to the max as well. A blended family of ADHD kids, who could ask for more? All my fears were abated when I realized we were all the same and in the same boat. I'll tell you more about this later. If you can afford it, some private schools offer smaller class sizes and individualized attention, which can benefit students with ADHD.

Understanding Vouchers

Vouchers can provide some families, "when offered," the financial means to access private children's education or specialized schools that might better meet their child's child's needs. Researching the availability and eligibility requirements for school vouchers in your area is essential, as they vary. Vouchers were unavailable when I raised my children in the '80s and '90s. The last two children were in the 2000s, but where we lived, vouchers were unavailable.

Evaluating Your Child's Needs

Consider your child's specific challenges with ADHD and learning style when exploring educational options. Consult with educational professionals, therapists, or other parents of children with ADHD for insights and advice. I would advise you to look at homeschooling or a homeschooling-type model where they have access to teachers through computers, But not the influence of dysfunctional children in the public school system, *which they tend to gravitate to with ADHD*. If they're struggling in the public school system, try homeschooling at least through the elementary grades, where children's impressions are great. I know you, maybe thinking this guy is crazy, we can't do that. We both have to work to survive. Yes, the American dream is becoming increasingly challenging to acquire. Parents are working three jobs. It's ridiculous. One of our daughters works for a company that handles complaints and other customer issues. This was because she couldn't afford childcare for her children and make a living. I don't know how she does it, having people screaming in her ear and two children climbing all over her, but she does it. I have remarkable daughters as well. I am not bragging, just saying.

Another option, I know, is not for everyone running your own business. That's the one we chose before starting our business. We both worked outside the home. My wife worked nights at the hospital as a nurse. She worked three 12-hour days and was paid for 40 hours, Friday, Saturday, and Sunday every week.

On the other hand, I worked Monday through Thursday, 10-hour days. You may think we were just fortunate, but it took a lot of negotiations to get this in place. We had to miss every weekend together. After doing this for years, we decided to start our own business, as our company became more successful. We both were able to leave our jobs and work there. Our children, who pitched in, saw us in our roles working hard, which shaped their work ethic. It was, I think, some of the best years of all of our lives. Our 2 ADHD boys did marketing and deliveries. I saw them go from being nonsocial, one more than the other, to being very personable and effective. Unfortunately, in 2018, after 13 years in business, after four spinal surgeries, my inability to work effectively, as I became more and more disabled, and due to cuts in government contracts, we had to close the business. I'd have to write another book to tell you about everything that happened, but to sum it up, it was a very blessed time in our lives working with our children. It's worth it.

Balancing Academic and Emotional Needs

Academic Environment and Emotional Well-being: Choose an educational environment that addresses academic needs and supports your child's emotional and social development. For children with ADHD, traditional schooling may not always be the most effective path. Homeschooling, school choice, and vouchers offer alternative options tailored to these children's needs. Each option has its own set of benefits and challenges, and the children should be based on a careful evaluation of the child's individual needs and family circumstances. By considering these alternatives, parents can make informed decisions that enhance their child's educational experience and overall development. In the following chapters, we will delve into strategies for academic success within these various educational settings and how to integrate the chosen approach with the overall management of ADHD. When both parents work outside the home, sometimes it isn't worth it if your children aren't getting the love, time, and education they need. Consider making some concessions now for their education, smaller home, used car, whatever it takes to allow you to build that child-parent connection, and be the person they spend the most time with and, by example, imitate.

Utilizing Public and Government Educational Resources

Government and Educational Websites

- U.S. Department of Education: Access resources provided by the U.S. Department of Education (www.ed.gov) for information on educational policies, programs, and assistance.

- National Center for Learning Disabilities: Visit websites like the National Center for Learning Disabilities (www.ncld.org) for strategies and resources specifically tailored for children with learning challenges.

Online Public Education Platforms

- Khan Academy: Utilize platforms like Khan Academy (www.khanacademy.org) for free educational resources across various subjects.

- Public Library Resources: Explore online resources offered by public libraries, which often include access to educational materials, tutoring services, and interactive learning activities.

As of my last update in April 2023, the National Center for Education Statistics (NCES) noted approximately 3% to 4% of school-age children in the United States were homeschooled before the COVID-19 pandemic. However, this percentage saw a significant increase during the pandemic. According to data from the U.S. Census Bureau's Household Pulse Survey, the rate of homeschooling (not including virtual learning through public or private schools) rose to around 5.4% by the start of the 2020-2021 school year. Then, it increased to approximately 11% by the fall of 2020. So, pandemic data was bad news for local schools, but I know it didn't stay at that level.

Furthermore, the Household Pulse Survey conducted by the

U.S. Census Bureau provides additional insight into the homeschooling trend, revealing that by May 2023, 85% of students were enrolled in public schools, 9.6% attended private schools, and 5.4% were homeschooled. This data suggests that the rate of homeschooling had stabilized at around 5.4% following a substantial increase from pre-pandemic levels when only 2.8% of students were reported as being homeschooled in 2019 . Don't you love data? (Not the guy in Star Trek), However, a plethora of information can be found online.

Balancing Spiritual and Public Educational Perspectives

Harmonizing Faith and Academic learning, someone listens. Strive to integrate your spiritual teachings with academic knowledge, ensuring your child receives a well-rounded education. Teach your child to apply critical thinking and discernment, balancing faith-based learning with general theoretical understanding.

The Role of the Spiritual Leader and Worship Family in Educational Support Spiritual Guidance and Support

- spiritual leader Counseling: Seek spiritual leader counseling for guidance on integrating Godly values into your child's education and for support in addressing any challenges.

- Prayer and Spiritual Support: Request prayers and spiritual support from your place of worship community. The power of collective prayer and encouragement can be a source of strength and comfort in a place of worship.

Educational Programs

Utilize places of worship and educational programs, like Sunday school or Bible study classes, as supplementary educational resources that provide spiritual nurturing. Encourage participation in youth group activities, which can offer additional learning opportunities and social interaction.

Involvement of the Place of Worship in Educational Development

Mentorship and Tutoring

- place of worship-Based Tutoring: Some congregations offer tutoring programs. These can be valuable resources, mainly if they include members who are educators or have experience with ADHD.

- Mentorship Programs: Engage with place of worship mentorship programs where older congregation members mentor younger ones, providing guidance and support in academic and spiritual matters. We found this helpful, especially since our place of worship was essential as an extended family.

Community Learning Opportunities

- Educational Workshops and Seminars: Participate in educational workshops or seminars offered by the place of worship. These can cover various topics, including parenting strategies, child development, and learning techniques.

- Volunteer and Service Projects: Involve your child in place of worship volunteer and service projects. These activities can provide practical learning experiences and help develop a sense of responsibility and community.

Integrating place of worship and Home Educational Efforts

Consistent Messaging and Support

- Aligning place of worship Teachings with Home Education: Ensure that the teachings and values imparted at the place of prayer align with those reinforced at home. Consistency in messaging helps in the overall development of the child.

- Regular Communication with the Place of Worship Leaders: Maintain open lines of communication with the worship leaders about your child's progress and educational challenges. This enables them to provide more tailored support.

The spiritual leader, congregation, parish, and other places of worship can play a significant role in the educational support system for a child with ADHD. Their involvement extends beyond spiritual guidance, offering emotional support, mentorship, and practical learning opportunities. By integrating the resources and support of the place of worship community with home-based educational efforts, parents can create a comprehensive support system that nurtures the child's academic, spiritual, and personal growth. In the upcoming chapters, we will discuss extending this integrated approach to broader social interactions and preparing for transitions in the child's academic and spiritual journey.

Enhancing learning at home for a child with ADHD can be a holistic process incorporating Faith principles and public educational resources. By blending these perspectives, you can provide a comprehensive educational experience that caters to your child's child's spiritual and academic growth. This approach supports their learning needs and helps nurture a well-rounded individual grounded in faith and knowledge.

In the following chapters, we will explore further strategies for facilitating social development and preparing for future educational transitions within a balanced spiritual and public education framework.

Chapter Thirteen

Make a Difference with Your Review (I hope)

Mid-Book Review Request Page

Real-Life Impact: ADHD basketball debacle

A poignant example of how ADHD symptoms can escalate occurred during a basketball game involving my son. His inability to control his impulses led to an aggressive outburst on the basketball court, suspending him. This incident was a stark reminder of how ADHD can impact not just academic but also social and extracurricular activities. After he was pulled from that game, getting along with the other boys on the team became very d-ifficult, leading him to no longer want to play. It was regrettable for him and all of us. He was outstanding. I felt he could have played college ball. This broke my heart for him. I wish I could have forced him to return to the team, but it was impossible after speaking to his coach, who said he couldn't manage his behavior. ADHD in the 1980s was not well understood, but at first, I felt I wanted to punch his coach. But that would set us a bad example and have beaten me up. He was a huge guy. I was just being honest, as I said earlier in this book.

> "We cannot always build the future for our youth, but we can make our youth for the future.
> **Franklin D. Roosevelt**:

People who give without expectation live longer, happier lives and make more money. So if we've got a shot at that during our time together, darn it, I'm going to try. To make that happen, I have a question for you...

Would you help someone you've never met, even if you never got credit for it?

Who is this person you ask? They are like you. Or, at least, like you used to be. Less experienced, wanting to make a difference, and needing help, but unsure where to look.

Our mission is to make this parents' guide accessible to everyone. Everything We do stems from that mission. And, the only way for Us to accomplish that mission is by reaching...well...everyone. OK, almost everyone in the world.

This is where you come in. Most people judge a book by its cover (and its reviews). So here's my ask on behalf of a struggling Parent of a Son with ADHD

Please help that struggling parent by leaving a review of this book.

Your gift costs no money and takes less than 60 seconds to make real, but it can change the life of a fellow parent of an ADHD boy forever. Your review could help...

...one more Parent transforms their life.

...one more Boy's dream come true.

To get that 'feel good' feeling and help this person for real, all you have to do is...and it takes less than 60 seconds...

Leave a review.

Scan the QR code below to leave your review:

[https://www.amazon.com/review/review-your-purchases/?asin=BOOKASIN]

If you feel good about helping faceless Parents, you are my kind of person. Welcome to the club. You're one of us.

I'm much more excited to help you Reach other Parents than you could imagine. You'll love the Humor and a plethora of information I'm about to share in the coming chapters.

Thank you from the bottom of my heart. Now, back to our regularly scheduled programming.

- Your biggest fan, Patrick J Steadman

PS - Fun fact: If you provide something of value to another person, it makes you more valuable to them. If you'd like good-will straight from another parent and believe this book will help them, send it their way.

Chapter Fourteen

Fostering Social Skills and Friendships

This chapter addresses the crucial aspect of social development for children with ADHD. Social skills and nurturing friendships are vital for their emotional and social well-being. We will explore strategies to help overcome social challenges and encourage positive peer interactions.

Overcoming Social Challenges

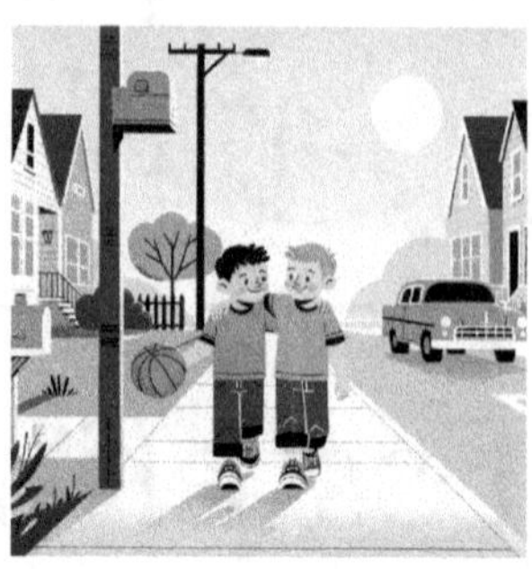

Children with ADHD often face unique social challenges due to difficulties with impulsivity, hyperactivity, and interpreting social cues.

Understanding Social Difficulties

Teach your child to understand and empathize with others' feelings. This can be done through discussions, stories, and role-playing exercises. Have you ever gone out to dinner with someone who didn't close your mouth when they chewed? I had a friend We went out to dinner with, and afterward, I almost felt defiled food falling out of his mouth, chewing so loud that you could hear him 10 feet away. We were still friends, but I never went to dinner with them again. His children ate the same way, like going to dinner with cattle. Consider enrolling your child in social skills training programs, which can provide structured guidance in understanding social norms and behaviors.

Building Confidence in Social Situations

Start with small, manageable social interactions. Guide and support your child in these settings, gradually helping them to build confidence. Acknowledge and praise your child's efforts in social interactions, even the small steps, to reinforce positive social behavior. Waiting their turn in line, allowing other kids to go before them, and showing kindness, please, thank you. These, and many different social reactions, will teach good behavior and acceptance in social settings. Where they're congratulated for good social behavior and manners, engage your child in activities where they feel comfortable and can succeed, such as structured group activities or interest-based clubs. Arrange playdates or small group activities with peers who understand and support the child's needs.

Facilitating Peer Understanding

Support the child. With the child's consent, educate their peers about ADHD. This can foster understanding and reduce the likelihood of misunderstandings. 'Encourage siblings and family members to model inclusive behavior. Their acceptance can be influential in shaping peer interactions.

Navigating the Digital Social roadmap in today's digital age, social interactions often occur online. Navigating this digital social landscape can be particularly challenging for children with ADHD." Educate your child about online behavior, including what's appropriate to share and how to interact respectfully." Keep an eye on your child's online interactions, ensuring they are positive and safe." Today, many different applications can monitor a child's online behavior and communicate that to you in real-time.

Faith Relationships and Social Development in the Worship Community

They are building Relationships within the Worship Community. Encourage participation in your place of worship youth groups, religious school classes, and other place of worship-related activities. These settings provide a safe and nurturing environment for developing social skills within a community with similar values. Seek out mentorship opportunities for your child within the place of worship. A mentor who understands how faith can provide guidance and a positive role model. They are forming relationships with those who share similar values and beliefs, especially in friendship and, later in life, romantic relationships. Guide your child in choosing friends who uplift and support their faith and values. This doesn't mean avoiding friendships outside the faith community but being mindful peers'rs' influence on each other.

Encouraging Inclusive and Supportive Peer Interactions

Advocate for an inclusive and accepting environment within the worship community. Encourage worship leaders and youth group coordinators to be aware of and accommodate the unique needs of children with ADHD. With your child's permission, consider opportunities to educate their peers about ADHD. Understanding can foster empathy and more robust, more supportive relationships.

Guidance on Peer Pressure and Choices

Equip your child with the skills to navigate peer pressure, especially in scenarios that may conflict with their values. Role-playing and discussions can be practical tools. Teach your child to make decisions based on your values and principles, reinforcing the importance of these values in shaping their actions and choices.

Integrating Faith relationships and principles in fostering social skills and friendships provides children with ADHD a strong foundation for their social development. By involving them in the place of worship, teaching them about forming relationships that align with their faith, and guiding them in inclusive and empathetic interactions, we can help them build meaningful and supportive relationships. This approach not only aids their social development but also strengthens their spiritual growth.

In the following chapters, we will explore how to translate these skills and values into other areas of life, such as school and community involvement, creating a well-rounded approach to social development. Fostering social skills and friendships in children with ADHD involves understanding their unique social challenges, creating positive social opportunities, and guiding them in in-person and online interactions. By supporting their social development in these ways, we can help them build meaningful relationships and enhance their overall social competence.

Understanding Bad or Destructive Relationships Relationships

Discuss the importance of forming relationships with those with similar values and beliefs, especially in friendship and, later in life, in romantic relationships. Guide your child in choosing friends who uplift and support their faith and values. That doesn't mean avoiding friendships outside the faith community but being mindful that peers influence each other.

Embracing the Friendship Ethic

Encourage your child to understand and practice the principle of 'be a friend to have a friend.' This involves showing kindness, understanding, and support to others, thereby building strong and meaningful friendships. Demonstrate how to be a good friend through your actions. This includes showing compassion, listening well, and offering help when needed. Ensure your child and you that though you're there for them and they're treating you poorly, this may be a toxic friendship. Not all relationships are worth keeping, so encourage them to look for positive relationships. Once, I used the adage on my daughter, "If your friends jump off of a Cliff, would you "jump off too?" "Well," she replied, "If I had "a parachute, I would." I know she got the point. At least, I think she did.

Teach your child to be welcoming and inclusive in their approach to making friends, reflecting humble acceptance of all people. Educate your child about embracing differences in others, whether cultural, social, or personal, that can enhance empathy and broaden their perspective.

> "Do not train a child to learn by force or harshness, but direct them to it by what amuses their minds so that you may be better able to discover with accuracy the peculiar bent of the the genius of each."
>
> Plato

Being 'Salt and Light' in Social Interactions

Influencing Others Positively

'Encourage your child to live out religious values in their "interactions, being an example of salt and light' as said in the bible, to their peers. This means bringing positivity, hope, and goodness into their social circles. "Guide your child in standing firm in their faith and values, even when faced with challenges or peer pressure. Involve your child in service and outreach activities through worship or community. This provides opportunities for social interaction and allows them to make a positive impact. Encourage your child to take on leadership roles in youth groups or community projects, fostering a "sense of responsibility and confidence.

> "It is easier to build strong children than to repair broken men."
>
> **Frederick Douglass**

Nurturing Social Skills through Spiritual Teachings

Applying Scriptual Lessons to Everyday Life

Use stories and parables from the spiritual teachings to illustrate lessons about friendship, kindness, and making a positive impact. Or other literature From your place of worship or even secular groups in men and women of the past. Encourage regular prayer and reflection on their interactions and relationships, seeking guidance and wisdom from their spiritual groups.

Integrating faith values and teachings into the development of social skills and friendships can have a profound impact on children with ADHD. By embracing the principles of being a friend to have a friend and being 'salt and light' in the world, they can learn to form healthy, positive, and lasting relationships. These principles guide them in their social interactions and strengthen their spiritual journey.

<u>Family Recreation and Hobbies:</u>

Dedicate time to hobbies or crafts that relax and fulfill you. These activities can be therapeutic, whether painting, gardening, or playing an instrument. I play guitar, which I've done since I was 12. It is a great pleasure for me. I may not be the best guitarist, but I'm not the worst, I hope. My hands don't work as well as they used to. I did get an injection in my thumbs today, which hurt, by the way. But I highly recommend it. I'm able to move my thumbs around without a lot of pain. He said my thumb moved from the joint to the right, hoping it wouldn't fall off. Why am I telling you about my thumbs? That's my ADHD. Let's move on. I also love to paint animals and people's pets; I would paint a pet and get a small royalty. No, it barely covered the cost of the paint and canvas I used. It's like free painting, so become an amateur at something and enjoy it. Again, I'm so sorry; let's move on.

A Personal Journey without Discovery

Plan regular family recreational activities that are relaxing and enjoyable for everyone. This could be anything from movie nights to board game sessions. My children are grown now, as I'm 63; I became disabled at 58 due to a botched surgery. My wife and I spent time at the rec center and on stationary bikes in our 40s. I'd rather be doing something productive, like building something or doing anything else. I didn't get this stationary bike thing; I felt like I should be manufacturing electricity or something. I did run in my 50s, nine or so miles a week. The endorphins were terrific, but my back and knees began to hate me for it. Now I walk like Quasimodo, dragging a leg. Okay, well, that's enough whining from me. Find out what your happy place is. And get out and do it.

Integrating Mindfulness into Your Routine

Adopt a mindful approach to parenting. This means being present at the moment with your child, actively listening to them, and engaging with them without the distraction of other thoughts or stressors. Mindfully r-eflect on your day and interactions with your child. This can help in understanding and managing your reactions and responses better.

Mindfulness Techniques

- Daily Meditation or Prayer: Incorporate short daily sessions into your routine. Even a few minutes can help clear the mind and reduce stress.

- Mindful Breathing: Utilize mindful breathing techniques, especially during high stress, to help regain a sense of calm and control.

Parenting Support Groups

Join parenting support groups, especially those focused on ADHD. Sharing experiences and learning from other parents can be incredibly helpful. Engage with online forums or communities for additional support and resources. If you type 'ADHD forum or community, you'll see several pops up. These platforms can provide valuable advice and a sense of solidarity. It also allows you to meet other families and their children and find out just how screwed up they are. This can make you feel better in a twisted sort of way. I'm kidding. Have you ever vis-

ited somebody's home, and their children are so perfect you throw up a little in your mouth? You become good friends with them so that you can discover something wrong to make you feel better. Some people are better at this than others, but you be you. Look at your successes. Focus on what others do well to incorporate into Kids' lives. Share your own experiences and strategies with other parents. Offering support can also be a way of reinforcing your coping strategies and can provide a sense of fulfillment.

Reducing stress as a parent of a child with ADHD involves a holistic approach that includes personal care, mindfulness practices, physical and creative activities, and engaging with support groups. By implementing these strategies, you can manage your stress more effectively and create a more positive and nurturing environment for your family. Remember, taking care of your well-being is integral to being your best parent.

The following chapters will explore strategies for extending these principles, navigating the healthcare roadmap, and embracing your particular journey.

Chapter Fifteen

Navigating Healthcare and Professional Services Understanding Healthcare Options

Professional Services

This chapter is dedicated to exploring the importance of finding and building a supportive community and effectively navigating healthcare and professional services for parents of children with ADHD. Establishing a network of support and knowing how to access and utilize professional services can significantly ease the challenges associated with managing ADHD. In my former life, I did billing using billing codes. We have advanced considerably today, leading to ICD10 codes and adding more confusion. Physicians and other entities use these codes to identify diagnoses. The diagnosis codes for Attention-Deficit/Hyperactivity Disorder (ADHD) are found in the International Classification of Diseases (ICD), a global standard for reporting diseases and health conditions. As of my last update in April 2023, the ICD-10 (10th revision) is widely used, though some countries may have transitioned to ICD-11.

In the ICD-10, the codes for ADHD are:

1. **F90.0** - Disturbance of activity and attention: This code is used for the typical form of ADHD, which includes symptoms of inattention, hyperactivity, and impulsivity.

2. **F90.1** - Hyperkinetic conduct disorder: This code is used when ADHD symptoms are accompanied by conduct disorder.

3. **F90.8** - Other hyperkinetic disorders: This is for ADHD-like disorders that don't fit into other categories.

4. **F90.9** - Hyperkinetic disorder, unspecified: This code is used when diagnosing ADHD but does not specify a subtype.

The codes above were provided here for

Get to know your child's teachers and ensure they know you; like Mama Bear would say, "he has ADHD." Let's get this right. Metaphorically, putting on her mother Shirly's shoes before she goes to dialogue with his teachers usually means she is ready for a fight. If you are always prepared for a fight, you'll find one. I hope she doesn't read this. Anyway, her dying love and defense of her children did get some things done at the school to help her manage his ADHD. Some teachers don't seem to understand that it's not all his fault.

Building Your Community

Actively participate in events, workshops, and seminars related to ADHD. This increases your knowledge and helps you connect with other parents and professionals. Volunteer in ADHD awareness programs or community events. This can help build a supportive network and raise awareness abo ADHD. My wife being an RN meant she was pretty well versed in mental disorders, and having raised our kids made us quasi-experts, we thought. Even today, you sometimes want to shake them as adults and say, "What were you thinking"? Maintain regular consultations with healthcare professionals specializing in ADHD, including pediatricians, psychiatrists, and therapists. Encourage adult children to seek counseling because we don't always have the answers. When you feel you learned as much as possible about ADHD, and there's still much more to learn. Not me, but everyone else, though, kidding. Could you not give me a bad review? Stay informed about the latest treatments and therapies for ADHD. This includes medication, behavioral therapy, and alternative treatments.

Accessing Professional Services

Utilize the expertise of educational psychologists and counselors for personalized strategies to support your child's learning and emotional needs. Consider therapy sessions with behavioral specialists who can offer tailored strategies for managing ADHD symptoms. Don't be afraid they will lock you up after meeting you, maybe me, but not the reader; five stars in my review if you please.

Leveraging Community and Online Resources

Utilizing Online Platforms

Use educational websites and forums to access resources, research studies, and connect with experts in ADHD. This was never available to us as we raised our kids in the '80s and '90s, but I like that concept. My daughter is a nursing student; the last kid is still at home and was diagnosed in the previous year with ADHD. She had so much trouble organizing. We've tried and tried, but no matter what we did, we could not get her organized. She took herself to the doctor. She struggles with weight gain; we thought it might have been related to something else. Surely not ADHD. But her life changed when she started on medication. Attend and participate in online learning courses to deepen her and our renewed understanding of ADHD management. After having two boys with it, you would think we would recognize the signs and symptoms. Type free ADHD courses online and choose something. You won't even have to leave the house. That's not the only reason I like it, but it's one.

Community Programs and Resources

If possible, attend workshops and seminars on ADHD at local hospitals, schools, or community centers. Please work with your child's school to access resources they may offer, such as counseling services or special education programs. Trying this could be difficult, but let's return to the online stuff.

Integrating Community Support into Daily Life

Regular Engagement with Support Groups

Make regular participation in support groups a part of your routine. These groups can provide ongoing support, practical advice, and emotional comfort. Actively share your experiences and learn from group members how challenging their kids are. Then again, you can walk away feeling superior, having read this book. I'm kidding; I'm sure other books are just as informative, not. This reciprocal exchange can provide new insights and coping strategies.

Navigating Healthcare and Professional Services Effectively

Maintaining Strong Communication with Healthcare Providers

Maintain an open and ongoing dialogue with your child's healthcare providers. Keep them informed about your child's progress and any concerns you may have. Be proactive in seeking information about new treatments, therapies, and management techniques for ADHD.

Utilizing Professional Services

If applicable, ensure regular therapy sessions for your child to help them develop coping mechanisms and behavioral strategies. Educational Support Services: Explore educational support services, such as tutoring or special education programs, to support your child's academic needs.

Leveraging Online Resources and Technology

Educational and Supportive Online Platforms

Utilize web-based tools and resources that offer educational support, such as online tutoring or educational games tailored to children with ADHD. Engage with online forums and platforms for additional support. These can be a valuable source of information and connection with others. Online Research and Webinars: Regularly research the latest developments in ADHD management and attend webinars or online seminars. Consider digital health services, such as teletherapy or online consultations, for convenient access to healthcare professionals.

Note:

Integrating community support, healthcare resources, and online tools into your family's routine is crucial in managing your child's ADHD effectively. These resources provide valuable support, information, and practical strategies to enhance your child's well-being and development. By actively engaging with these resources and maintaining a proactive approach, you can ensure a holistic management plan that addresses all aspects of ADHD.

In the following chapters, we will explore strategies for ensuring long-term success and managing adolescent and adult life transitions for children with ADHD.

Chapter Sixteen

High-Risk Behaviors – Understanding and Addressing Drugs and ADHD

In this critical chapter, we address the sensitive yet vitally essential topics of high-risk behaviors, particularly drug abuse and suicide, in individuals with ADHD. Understanding these risks, recognizing the signs, and knowing how to respond effectively is essential for parents and caregivers.

Understanding the Risks

Increased Vulnerability to ADHD

- Statistical Insights: Research indicates that individuals with ADHD may have a higher propensity for engaging in high-risk behaviors, including substance abuse and suicidal tendencies.

- Factors Contributing to Risk: These risks can be attributed to impulsivity, a common symptom of ADHD, as well as potential coexisting conditions such as depression or anxiety.

Preventing Substance Abuse

Early Intervention and Education

Open Communication: Foster an environment where open and honest discussions about drug use are encouraged. Educate your child about the risks and consequences of substance abuse. Positive Coping Strategies: Teach and reinforce positive coping mechanisms for stress and emotional regulation as alternatives to substance use. In the complex parenting journey, especially during the teenage years, monitoring your child's well-being and guiding them through life's challenges are pivotal responsibilities. This includes being vigilant about the potential risks of substance abuse, a concern that can profoundly affect families. Here's how to approach monitoring and guidance effectively:

Stay Informed

Awareness is your first line of defense against substance abuse. Educating yourself on the signs and symptoms of drug use is crucial. These signs can be subtle or overt and may include changes in behavior, appearance, health, and social activities. Look out for sudden secrecy, withdrawal from family activities, changes in friends, or unexplained absences from school. Unexplained weight loss or gain, changes in sleep patterns, or deteriorating physical appearance. Mood swings, unexplained aggression, or symptoms of depression and anxiety. Academic or Professional Performance: Declining grades, loss of interest in school or extracurricular activities, or issues at work. Being informed also means understanding the substances that are commonly abused and the contexts in which abuse might occur. This knowledge can help you initiate open, non-judgmental conversations with your child about the dangers of drugs and alcohol.

Seek Professional Help

If you observe signs that suggest substance abuse, it's essential to act swiftly but calmly. Seeking professional help is a critical step. Early intervention can significantly affect the outcome for your child. Here are steps to consider: Consult a Healthcare Professional: Start with your family doctor, who can provide initial advice and referrals to specialists if necessary. Experts in substance abuse can offer comprehensive assessments and tailored intervention strategies. They can guide you and your child through recovery, offering medical and psychological support. Individual or family counseling can be invaluable. Therapists specialize in dealing with substance abuse and can help uncover underlying issues, such as stress, anxiety, or depression, that may contribute to the problem.

Foster an Open Environment

It is essential to create a supportive environment where your child feels safe to share their experiences and challenges without fear of judgment or harsh consequences. Open communication is vital to regularly talking about the risks and consequences of drug and alcohol use. Use current events or media stories as conversation starters. Please encourage your child to share their thoughts and feelings. Listen more than you speak to understand their perspective and build trust. Not Blame: Focus on expressing concern for your child's well-being rather than assigning blame. Make it clear that you're there to support and help them.

Be a Positive Role Model

Children often model their behavior on that of their parents. Demonstrating healthy coping mechanisms for stress, modeling responsible behavior regarding alcohol, and maintaining a substance-free lifestyle can significantly influence your child's choices. Well, and of course, not stabbing anyone in the leg or anywhere else. My parents consistently smoked and occasionally drank, mostly Schlitz, an excellent German beer. Not really; as I grew older, I found it disgusting. Anyway, on any Saturday or after school, you could find me, my brother, and my sister playing Margaret and Bill, played by my brother or me, with cigarette butts and empty beer cans. We have a grand performance, if not a little over the top. We usually ended up in a played argument where Margaret complained about Bill's drinking, and Bill complained about Margaret's smoking. As I look back at it now, it almost seems like child abuse. Regardless, it was usual for the day. I still miss them as they passed away in 2000 and 2004. First, my mother, then my father. Back to Business.

Monitor and Set Boundaries

While respecting your child's growing need for independence, setting and enforcing reasonable boundaries is essential. Know where your child is, who they are with, and what they do, especially during high-risk times. Setting clear rules and consequences regarding drug and alcohol use is also essential. Monitoring your child's activities and guiding them through the challenges of adolescence requires a delicate balance of vigilance, communication, and support. And if your children are playing the Bill and Margaret or Sue and Patrick show, maybe take stock of your life. However, seeing how they see you and how you're portrayed could be beneficial. You can guide your child through these formative years with care and understanding by staying informed, seeking professional help when necessary, and fostering a relationship built on trust and open dialogue. Substance abuse is a serious concern, but with the right approach, it can be navigated successfully.

Chapter Seventeen

ADHD and Understanding Suicide Risks

Research indicates that individuals with ADHD have a higher risk of suicidal ideation and attempts compared to those without ADHD. Studies suggest that this risk is multifactorial, stemming from the challenges and comorbidities associated with ADHD, such as depression, impulsivity, and low self-esteem.

Addressing the Risk of Suicide

Recognizing the Warning Signs

It's crucial to stay alert to any signs that may indicate your child is experiencing depression or harboring suicidal thoughts. In our journey, we noticed that children, especially those with ADHD, might become withdrawn or unusually quiet. They might pull away from activities they once enjoyed, exhibit significant mood changes, or express hopelessness.

Encouraging Open Conversations on Mental Health

It is essential to establish a space where your child can openly express their feelings and thoughts. Personally, I found this more challenging than my wife did, but the value of this effort became clear to me. By promoting honest communication, we gain insights into our children's concerns. This strengthens our bond with them and assures them of the support from their family and the broader circle of those involved in their care.

Navigating Mental Health Challenges

Our children experienced distressing thoughts. Checkups to Include mental health evaluations for your child's regular health visit, but thankfully, we were able to intervene in time. The fear of suicide is a profound concern shared by many parents, especially those with children diagnosed with ADHD. Often, seeking external support is necessary to provide the best care for our children. Finding the right words and actions that support without inadvertently causing harm is a delicate balance. The journey includes learning how to communicate effectively and when to seek professional help to navigate these complex emotional landscapes. Engage with mental health professionals if you have concerns about your child's mental well-being—regular Mental checkups. Various studies have shown that the rate of suicidal thoughts and behaviors is significantly higher in individuals with ADHD compared to the general population. For instance, a study published in the *Journal of Attention Disorders* reported that adolescents with ADHD are nearly <u>four times more likely to attempt suicide</u> than their peers without ADHD.

Contributing Factors

Many individuals with ADHD also struggle with other mental health conditions like depression, anxiety, or bipolar disorder, which can further increase the risk of suicidal thoughts and behaviors. The impulsivity component of ADHD can lead to riskier behaviors and, in some cases, may contribute to suicidal actions without extensive planning or forethought.

Prevention and Support Strategies

Early Intervention and Treatment: Timely and effective treatment of both ADHD and any coexisting mental health conditions is critical. This can include medication, therapy, and lifestyle changes. Regular monitoring by healthcare providers and support from family and friends is essential. Being vigilant about changes in mood, behavior, and verbal expressions related to self-harm is crucial. Raising awareness about the link between ADHD and increased suicide risk is essential. Educating families, educators, and individuals with ADHD about this risk can lead to earlier identification and intervention.

Seeking Professional Help

Regular consultations with mental health professionals who specialize in ADHD and comorbid conditions are crucial. They can provide tailored strategies for managing ADHD symptoms and associated mental health challenges. Having access to crisis intervention resources, such as suicide hotlines and emergency mental health services, is essential for immediate support in critical situations. Understanding the increased risk of suicide in individuals with ADHD calls for a comprehensive approach that includes education, early intervention, regular monitoring, and ongoing support. Families, educators, and healthcare providers need to work collaboratively to provide a supportive environment that addresses the unique challenges faced by individuals with ADHD.

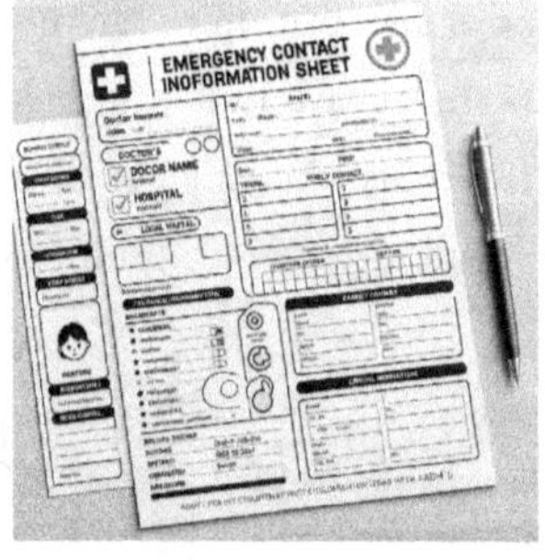

In our ongoing chapters, we will explore further the multifaceted approach needed to support individuals with ADHD across different stages of life, emphasizing the importance of a supportive community, continuous care, and the promotion of mental health and well-being.

Recent research indicates that individuals with ADHD, particularly adolescents and adults, are at an increased risk of suicidal spectrum behaviors (SSBs). A systematic review published in BMC Psychiatry in 2023 explored this connection, examining factors that may elevate the risk of SSBs in adults and adolescents with ADHD. The study identified several factors that increase the likelihood of SSBs, including ADHD symptom severity and persistence, female gender, family history of ADHD, childhood and parental influences, and social functioning. It was noted that even after adjusting for psychiatric comorbidities, individuals with ADHD still exhibit a heightened risk of SSBs. This review emphasizes the need for clinical implications in terms of screening and suicide prevention strategies, particularly in light of ADHD being an independent risk factor for SSBs.

In a separate study highlighted by The British Journal of Psychiatry, a cohort design using nationwide register data from Denmark was implemented to investigate whether individuals diagnosed with ADHD were more likely to exhibit suicidal behavior than those without ADHD. This study was notable for examining the role of psychiatric comorbid disorders in the association between ADHD and suicidality. The results showed a significantly higher incidence rate of suicidal behavior in individuals with ADHD compared to those without. The study found that males with ADHD had a 3.4-fold higher rate of suicidal behavior, whereas females with ADHD had a 9.1-fold higher rate compared to their counterparts without ADHD. This study highlights the critical need for early diagnosis and management of ADHD and co-occurring conditions to prevent elevated suicide risk and mortality.

These studies underscore the importance of recognizing the increased risk of suicide among individuals with ADHD and the necessity for comprehensive care and preventive strategies. You can refer to the articles in BMC Psychiatry and The British Journal of Psychiatry for more detailed information.

A journey of discovery and hope

In the journey of crafting this chapter, I was engulfed by the profound realities tied to the struggles with ADHD and the shadow of suicide. It's a heavy path to walk, a narrative filled with anguish and silent cries for help. Yet, amidst these trials, a beacon of hope emerges—a light assures us that despair does not mark the end.

To those who have felt the sting of loss, whose hearts have been shattered by suicide, I extend my deepest sympathies. The pain of losing a loved one in such a way is unimaginable, and it's a burden no one should bear alone.

But let's talk about where we go from here. In the face of such adversity, I've realized the immense power of discipline, accountability, and communication. It's not merely about teaching our children responsibility; it's about building a bridge of trust. A bridge that ensures they know, without a shadow of a doubt, that they can reach out to us in their darkest moments.

I want to share a story from my own life, a testament to the strength of this bond. My daughter, while not battling ADHD, faced her demons with depression—a struggle that is equally as life-threatening. There was a moment, heartbreakingly close to home, where she stood at the edge of a bridge, contemplating the end of a lost love. A love that, in the eyes of youth, seemed irreplaceable.

Yet, in that critical moment, the thought of her family's anguish gave her pause. She did something courageous; she called the police, fearing the impulse to leap might overtake her. The response was swift—a compassionate police officer, alongside her family, sat with her, talked through her pain, and helped her see that no heartache was worth her precious life. I thank God every day for that man and her safety.

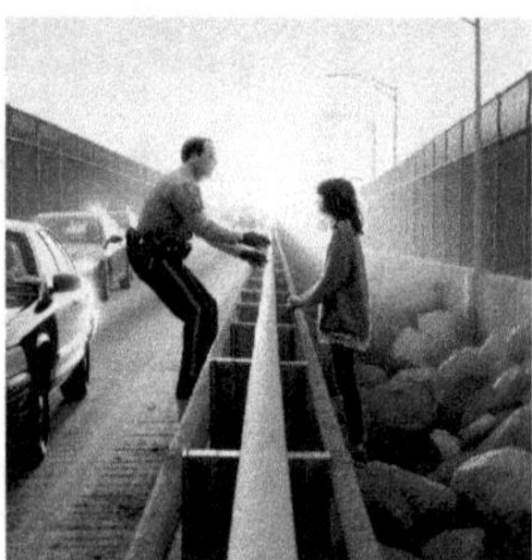

This experience underscored the vital importance of open communication. It's crucial to instill in our children the confidence to seek help when in need and to know that reaching out is not a sign of weakness but strength. While it's true that interactions with law enforcement can be daunting, a kind-hearted officer was a guardian angel in our case.

Today, my daughter lives joyfully, blessed with a loving husband and beautiful children. This journey has taught me that we can guide our children through the stormiest of seas through communication, understanding, and unconditional love. Let's pledge to be their beacon, ensuring they never feel alone in their struggles.

The study revealed a significant difference in the prevalence of suicide between patients with and without ADHD. The findings indicated a higher suicide rate among those with ADHD, underscoring a worrying reality. However, it was also noted that children with ADHD, when receiving proper medication and psychiatric care, have a lower risk of suicide. This aligns with my deepest fears about the potential for suicide in children with ADHD. We were lucky, but my heart goes to those less fortunate who have faced such tragedies. Despite close calls where our children expressed not wanting to live, we were able to intervene in time, preventing a tragic outcome.

Chapter Eighteen

Long-Term Strategies for Resilience and Well-being

Building a Supportive Environment Creating a Safe and Nurturing Home

S table and Supportive Home Environment: Strive to create a home environment that is stable, supportive, and understanding of your child's challenges. Encourage participation in activities that promote self-esteem, social interaction, and a sense of accomplishment.

Community and School Involvement

Leveraging Community Resources

Utilize community resources such as support groups, educational programs, and counseling services. Work closely with school counselors or psychologists to monitor your child's emotional and social well-being. Addressing high-risk behaviors such as drug abuse and suicide in children with ADHD requires vigilance, open communication, and proactive intervention. Understanding the risks, recognizing the signs, and having a response plan is vital to providing necessary support and intervention. Remember, you are not alone in this journey; resources and professionals are available to help guide and support you and your child.

Developing Emotional Resilience

Teach and reinforce emotional regulation skills. Techniques like mindfulness, deep breathing exercises, and cognitive-behavioral strategies can be instrumental. Focus on activities and opportunities that bolster self-esteem. Now we all know of the Little League team that gives everybody a trophy at the end of the year. Even though this seems a little ridiculous for young, impressionable children, it can be an esteem booster. But by the time my children reached the ages of seven and above, they expected recognition for actual competitive accomplishments, and no, your coloring book picture would not get into the Louvre. Celebrate successes, encourage efforts, and provide positive feedback on strengths and abilities.

Encouraging Healthy Relationships

Prioritize family time and activities that strengthen relationships and provide emotional security. Connections: Encourage friendships and social connections with peers with positive influences and shared interests.

Mental Health Professionals and Therapies

Maintain regular appointments with mental health professionals. Therapies, such as cognitive-behavioral therapy (CBT) or family therapy, can provide significant benefits. Be aware of and have access to crisis intervention resources, such as local crisis hotlines or emergency mental health services.

Educational and Community Support

Utilize school-based mental health programs and services. Regular communication with school counselors and teachers can help monitor and support the child's emotional health. Explore community mental health services and programs. These can include support groups, counseling services, and educational workshops.

Conclusion: Navigating the Healthcare System Advocating for Comprehensive Care

Preparing for the Future Equipping for Adulthood

Advocate for a holistic approach to your child's healthcare that considers physical and mental health. Ensure coordination between various healthcare providers for comprehensive care management, including pediatricians, psychiatrists, and therapists. Focus on life skills training as your child approaches adulthood. This includes skills for independent living, financial management, and employment readiness; our son Rich "remembers the boy stabbed in the leg by his new step-sister." Though my daughter thought He was a little irritating, stabbing him in the leg was probably a little over the top. She didn't hit anything vital. He was back to causing trouble in a day or two. Later, in his thirties, he studied plumbing, got a degree, and became a master plumber. He is now self-employed, running his own business. Work with healthcare providers and educators to develop a transition plan for adulthood, considering continuing education, employment, and independent living.

Tackling high-risk behaviors in children with ADHD presents a complex challenge that demands constant vigilance, all-encompassing support, and forward-thinking strategies. Parents play a crucial role in enhancing their child's safety, health, and future achievements by nurturing emotional resilience, fostering positive relationships, leveraging professional expertise, and planning for life's transitions.

The path of managing ADHD is ongoing, yet it can pave the way to a rewarding and prosperous existence with appropriate guidance and resources. In the chapters that follow, we will delve deeper into various facets of living with ADHD, such as transitioning into adulthood, leading a healthy lifestyle, and the importance of continuous advocacy and support. This includes reflecting on a critical moment when we faced the possibility of losing our daughter to suicide.

Addressing the sensitive topic of ADHD and its association with increased risks of suicide requires a careful and informed approach. Understanding the statistics and factors contributing to this increased risk and strategies for prevention and support is crucial.

Chapter Nineteen

Acknowledgements

- Reduced Symptoms of Inattention after Dietary Omega-3 Fatty Acid Supplementation in Boys with and without Attention Deficit/Hyperactivity Disorder Dienke J Bos et al. Neuropsychopharmacology. 2015 Sep.

- Urbano GL, Tablizo BJ, Moufarrej Y, Tablizo MA, Chen ML, Witmans M. The Link between Pediatric Obstructive Sleep Apnea (OSA) and Attention Deficit Hyperactivity Disorder (ADHD). Children (Basel). 2021 Sep 19;8(9):824. doi: 10.3390/children8090824. PMID: 34572256; PMCID: PMC8470037.

- O'Connor BC, Fabiano GA, Waschbusch DA, Belin PJ, Gnagy EM, Pelham WE, Greiner AR, Roemmich JN. Effects of a summer treatment program on functional sports outcomes in young children with ADHD. J Abnorm Child Psychol. 2014 Aug;42(6):1005-17. doi: 10.1007/s10802-013-9830-0. PMID: 24362766; PMCID: PMC4399495.

- Percentages of overdose deaths involving the most common opioids and stimulants alone or in combination[10] in 2022, *Overall (30 jurisdictions) CDC data 2022* SUDORS Dashboard: Fatal Overdose Data Final Data updated December 14, 2023; Preliminary Data updated December 14, 2023 Updated December 26, 2023

- Robert Myers Ph.D. Age-appropriate chores that work encouraging responsibility children .https://childdevelopmentinfo.com/chores/the-ultimate-list-of-age-appropriate-chores/

- U.S. Department of Education: Access resources provided by the U.S. Department of Education (www.ed.gov) for information on educational policies, programs, and assistance.

- National Center for Learning Disabilities: Visit websites like the National Center for Learning Disabilities (www.ncld.org) for strategies and resources specifically tailored for children with learning challenges.

- Staff AI, Oosterlaan J, van der Oord S, van den Hoofdakker BJ, Luman M. The Relation Between Classroom Setting and ADHD Behavior in Children With ADHD Compared to Typically Developing Peers. J Atten Disord. 2023 Jul;27(9):939-950. doi: 10.1177/10870547231167522. Epub 2023 Apr 11. PMID: 37039105; PMCID: PMC10291114. https://www.ncbi.nlm.nih.gov/pmc/articles/PMC10291114/#bibr21-10870547231167522

- Khan Academy is a 501(c)(3) nonprofit organization

- National Center for Education Statistics. (2022). Home-schooled Children and Reasons for Homeschooling. *Condition of Education*U.S. Department of Education, Institute of Education Sciences. Retrieved [date], from https://nces.ed.gov/programs/coe/indicator/tgk

- **CMS billing coding ICD-10 Implementation Date: October 1, 2015** Code services provided on or after Oct 1, 2015 with ICD-10

- **World Health Organization(WHO)** (1993). The ICD-10 classification of mental and behavioral disorders. World Health Organization.

- DALL-E GPT-4 used in imaging and editing

www.ingramcontent.com/pod-product-compliance
Lightning Source LLC
Chambersburg PA
CBHW070808260726
48660CB00005B/1773